AF413182

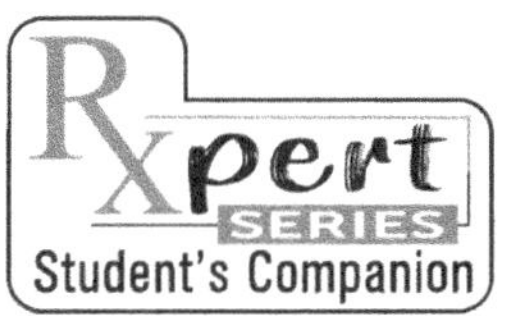

Pharmacognosy and Phytochemistry – II

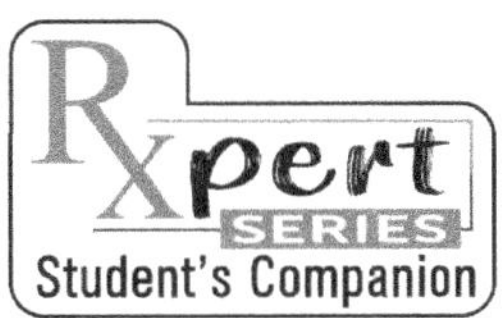

Pharmacognosy and Phytochemistry – II

Vishakha S Kulkarni

Professor

Department of Pharmacognosy

MNR College of Pharmacy

Sangareddy, Hyderabad

V. Alagarsamy

Professor & Principal

MNR College of Pharmacy

Sangareddy, Hyderabad

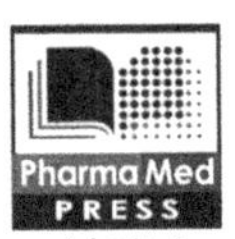

PharmaMed Press

An imprint of BSP Books pvt. Ltd

4-4-309/316, Giriraj Lane,

Sultan Bazar, Hyderabad - 500 095.

Pharmacognosy and Phytochemistry – II

by Vishakha S Kulkarni and V. Alagarsamy

Published by:

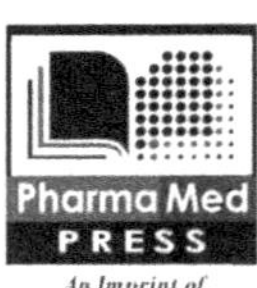

PharmaMed Press

An imprint of BSP Books Pvt. Ltd.

4-4-309/316, Giriraj Lane, Sultan Bazar, Hyderabad - 500 095.
Phone: 040-23445688; Fax: 91+40-23445611
e-mail: info@pharmamedpress.com
www.pharmamedpress.com/pharmamedpress.net

ISBN: 978-93-91910-23-5 (Hardack)

Preface

Pharmacognosy refers to the knowledge of drug substances (in Greek pharmakon- drug; gnosis- the knowledge). Pharmacognosy can be referred to as a scientific, which discipline is primarily concerned with the study of drugs obtained from natural sources such as plants, minerals and animals. Similarly, phytochemistry is a branch, which deal with the chemistry of the plant and plant products. The subject pharmacognosy and phytochemistry obviously deal with study of natural products and chemistry of the plants and plant-derived products. Recent trends in pharmacognosy and phytochemistryinvolveidentification, isolation and characterization of naturally occurring substances with the help of different analytical techniques.

The subject Pharmacognosy and phytochemistry-II extends the basic understanding of chemistry of plants or plant-derived products as well as methods of extraction, identification, isolation and estimation. The subject also emphasizes different analytical techniques used in analysis of phytoconstituents.

As the new syllabus by Pharmacy Council of India (PCI) is being implemented from 2017-18, we have taken opportunity to bring out this book on the title of "Pharmacognosy and Phytochemistry-II" As per PCI Revised B.Pharm Syllabus of Semester V; the third year B. Pharmacy. In this text earnest attempt has been made to describe the course content in accordance with the revised syllabus prescribed by PCI.

The book has covered the entire syllabus of Pharmacognosy and Phytochemistry II unit wise. At the beginning of every chapter/unit the syllabus for a particular unit is given followed by detailed description of topics. At the end of every unit attempt has been made to provide probable questionnaire. Designingtext sufficient care has been taken to provide suitable examples and figures/block diagram wherever applicable. The natural plant drug images have been given for better understanding and identification of the crude drugs.

In this book Unit I deal with basic metabolic pathways involved in the biosynthesis of secondary metabolites and the techniques used to determine the secondary metabolites in higher plants. Unit II describes representative crude drugs containing secondary metabolite as a chief chemical constituent like alkaloids, phenylpropanoids, flavonoids, steroids, cardiac glycosides, triterpenoids, volatile oils, tannins, resins, glycosides, irridoids, terpenoids, naphthaquinones and carotenoids. Unit III explains the methods of isolation, identification tests and estimation methods of important phytoconstituents. Similarly, Unit IV deals with commercial production methods, estimation methods and commercial applications of important phytoconstituents. Unit V explains the basics of phytochemistry and modern analytical techniques used in isolation, purification and identification of crude drugs and phytoconstituents like extraction methods, chromatographic techniques, spectroscopic methods and electrophoresis.

The text in the book is explained in a simple language with atmost care to cover each and every point of the syllabus. We hope that **"Pharmacognosy and Phytochemistry-II"** will be found more useful to fulfilllthe requirements of B. Pharmacy students.

- Authors

Contents

Unit IV

Industrial Production, Estimation and Utilization of Phytoconstituents

Unit V

Basics of Phytochemistry

Unit I

Metabolic Pathways in Higher Plants and their Determination

PCI Syllabus

Metabolic pathways in higher plants and their determination

- Brief study of basic metabolic pathways and formation of different secondary metabolites through these pathways- Shikimic acid pathway, Acetate pathways and Amino acid pathway.

- Study of utilization of radioactive isotopes in the investigation of Biogenetic studies

Book Chapter Content

- Introduction
- Basic Metabolic Pathways in Plants
- Shikimic Acid Pathway
- Biosynthesis of Amino Acids
- Acetate – Mevalonate Pathway
- Acetate Malonate Pathway
- Biosynthesis of Secondary Metabolites
  - Biosynthesis of Glycosides
  - Biosynthesis of Alkaloids
  - Biosynthesis of Isoprenoid Compounds
  - Biosynthesis of Triglycerides
  - Biosynthesis of Phenolic Compounds
- Stress Compounds
- Study of Utilization of Radioactive Isotopes in The Investigation of Biogenetic Studies
  - Tracer Techniques
  - Other Techniques to Investigate Biosynthetic Pathways

Introduction

Plant metabolism: It is defined as the complex physical and chemical events of photosynthesis, respiration, synthesis and degradation of organic compounds. Plant body is considered as a best biosynthetic laboratory than animal body for production of primary metabolites like sugars, amino acids and many secondary metabolites of pharmaceutical importance like glycosides, alkaloids, flavonoids, volatile oils, tannins, resins, enzymes, terpenes, color pigments etc.

Metabolism is considered as a sum of all biochemical processes and is distinguished into primary metabolism and secondary metabolism. The **primary metabolism** comprises of all the pathways necessary for survival of the cells, example photosynthesis, Calvin cycle, glycolysis, gluconeogenesis, Kreb's cycle etc.

Secondary metabolism produces a large number of specialized compounds (estimated around 200,000) which do not interfere in the growth and development of plants but are required for the plant to survive in its environment. Secondary metabolism is connected to primary metabolism by using building blocks and biosynthetic enzymes derived from primary metabolism. Primary metabolism governs all basic physiological processes that allow a plant to grow and set seeds, by translating the genetic code into proteins, carbohydrates, and amino acids. Specialized compounds from secondary metabolism are essential for communicating with other organisms through mutualistic (e.g. attraction of beneficial organisms such as pollinators) or antagonistic interactions (e.g. deterrent against herbivores and pathogens). They further assist in coping with abiotic stress such as increased UV-radiation. In any case, a good balance between products of primary and secondary metabolism is best for a plant's optimal growth and development as well as for its adjustment with often changing environmental conditions. Well known secondary metabolic compounds include alkaloids, glycosides, flavonoids, terpenoids etc. Humans use quite a lot of these compounds, or the plants from which they originate, for culinary, medicinal and nutraceutical purposes.

This unit comprises of overview of basic metabolic pathways and details about the secondary metabolites synthesis in plants.

Basic Metabolic Pathways in Plants

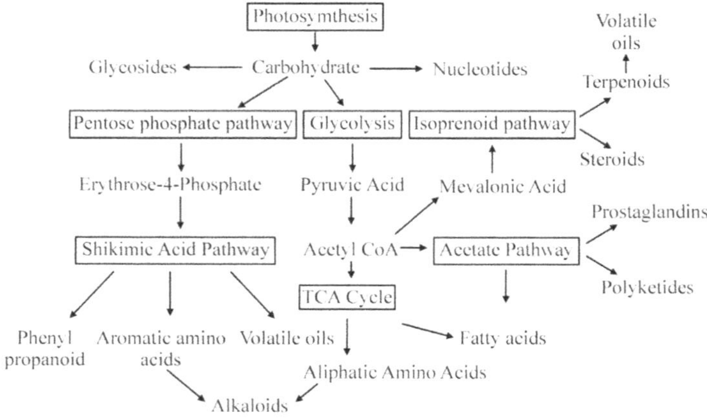

Fig. 1.1 Overview of biosynthesis of primary and secondary metabolites in plants

The products or byproducts of primary metabolism like carbohydrates, Acetyl COA, Shikimic acid and Mevalonic acid are used as building block or precursor for biosynthesis of secondary metabolites like alkaloids, glycosides, isoprenoids and many more. The important metabolic pathways are described here.

Shikimic Acid Pathway/Shikimate Pathway

The Shikimic acid pathway is a seven step metabolic pathway used by bacteria, archea, algae, fungi, some protozoans and plants for the biosynthesis of folates and aromatic amino acids *viz.* phenylalanine, tyrosine and tryptophan. This pathway is not found in animals and humans. Animlas and humans require these amino acids, hence the products of this pathway represents essential amino acids. The important steps involved in shikimic acid pathway are given below.

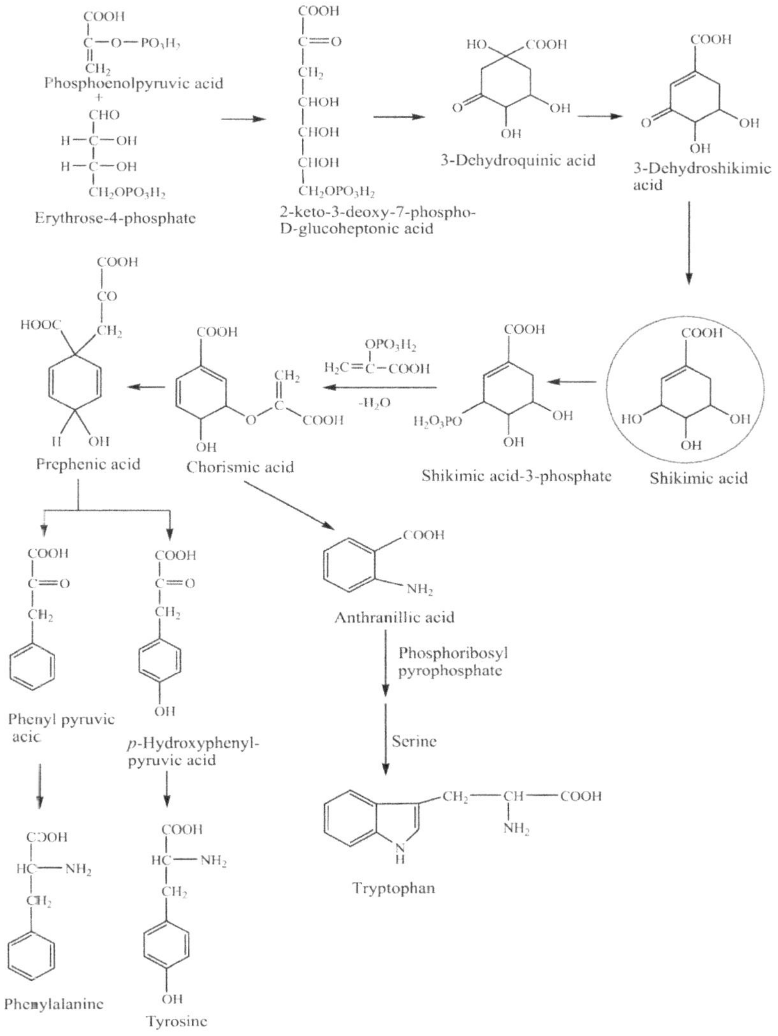

Fig 1.2 Shikimic acid pathway

Steps in Shikimic acid pathway

- Phosphoenolpyruvic acid and erythrose-4-phosphate react to form 2-keto-3-deoxy-7-phosphoglucoheptonic acid, in a reaction catalyzed by the enzyme *DAHP synthase.*

  2-keto-3-deoxy-7-phosphoglucoheptonic acid is then transformed to 3-dehydroquinic acid in a reaction catalyzed by *DHQ synthase.*

  Although this reaction requires nicotinamide adenine dinucleotide (NAD) as a cofactor, the enzymatic mechanism regenerates it, resulting in no net use of NAD.

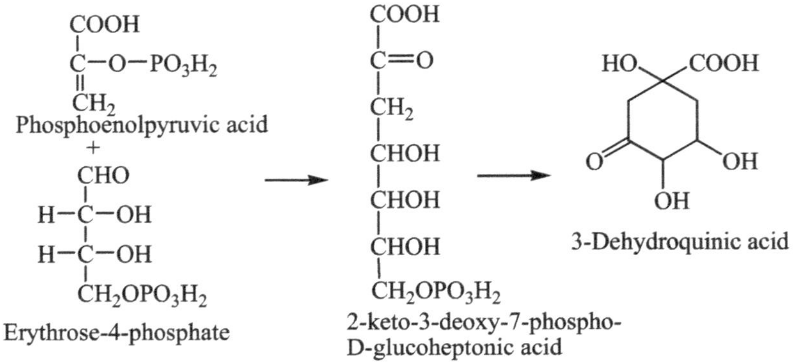

- 3-Dehydroquinic acid is dehydrated to 3-Dehydroshikimic acid by the enzyme 3-Dehydroquinate dehydratase, which is reduced to shikimic acid by the enzyme Shikimate dehydrogenase, which uses nicotinamide adenine dinucleotide phosphate (NADPH) as a cofactor.

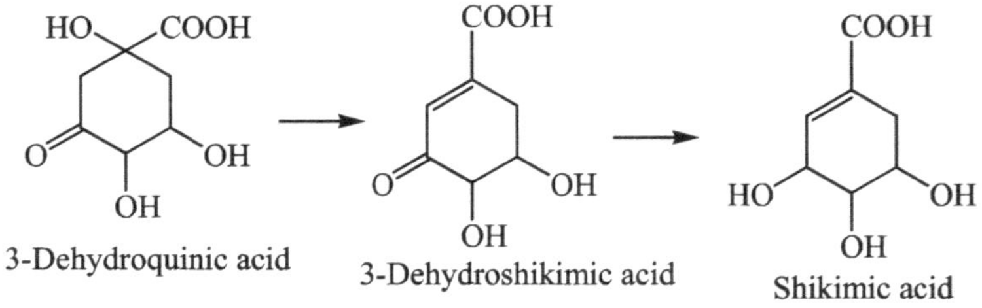

- The next enzyme involved is Shikimate kinase, an enzyme that catalyzes the ATP dependent phosphorylation of shikimic acid to form shikimate 3-phosphate. Shikimic acid 3-phosphate is then coupled with phosphoenol pyruvate to give 5-enolpyruvylshikimate-3-phosphate via the enzyme 5-enolpyruvylshikimate-3-phosphate (EPSP) synthase.

  Then 5-enolpyruvylshikimate-3-phosphate is transformed into chorismic acid by a chorismate synthase.

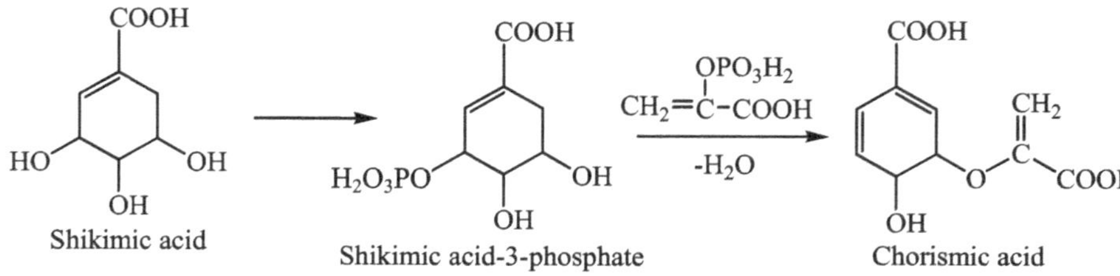

The formation of chorismic acid is the important step in the shikimic acid pathway as this compound can synthesize different types of intermediates.

- Prephenic acid is then synthesized by a Claisen rearrangement of chorismate by Chorismate mutase. The aromatic amino acids tyrosine and phenyl alanine are biosynthesized from prephenic acid   through independent pathways.

- Prephenic acid is oxidatively decarboxylated with retention of the hydroxyl group by prephenate dehydrogenase to give p-hydroxyphenylpyruvic acid, which is transaminated using glutamate as the nitrogen source to give tyrosine and α-ketoglutarate.

- Similarly, prephenic acid undergoes aromatization to synthesize phenyl pyruvic acid followed by reductive transamination to synthesize phenyl alanine.

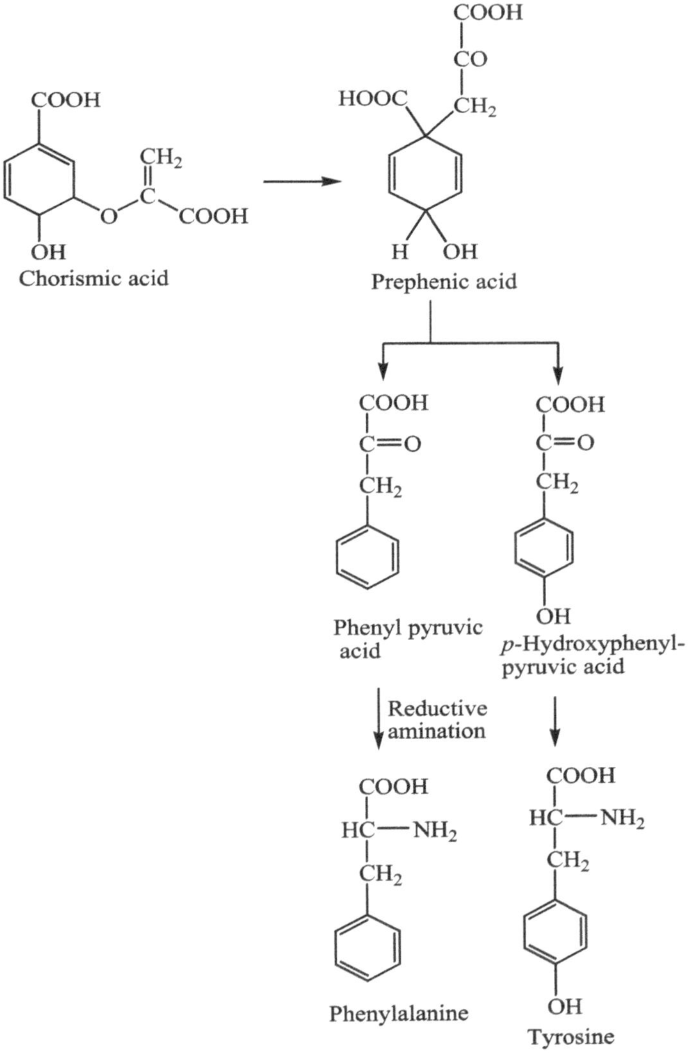

Chorismic acid

Prephenic acid

Phenyl pyruvic acid

p-Hydroxyphenyl-pyruvic acid

Reductive amination

Phenylalanine

Tyrosine

- In presence of glutamine, chorismic acid is converted to anthranilic acid. Later in conjugation with serine in presence of tryptophan synthase it converts into aromatic amino acid **Tryptophan**.

Chorismic acid → Anthranillic acid → (Phosphoribosyl pyrophosphate, serine) → Tryptophan

Importance of Shikimic Acid Pathway

Shikimic acid is a starting point of in the biosynthesis of some important secondary metabolites, as mentioned in the following examples.

1. Biosynthesis of glycosides *viz.*
   - (a) Cyanogenetic glycosides- Prunacin, amygdalin
   - (b) Isothiocyanate glycosides- Sinigrin
   - (c) Coumarin Glycosides- Psoralen
   - (d) Flavanoid glycoside- Quercetin, hesperidin
2. Biosynthesis of Alkaloids
   - (a) Alkaloids derived from Tryptophan- Physostigmine, quinine
   - (b) Alkaloids derived from Phenyl alanine, tyrosine and related amino acids- Ephedrine, papaverine etc.
3. Biosynthesis of lignin- Podophyllotoxin
4. Biosynthesis of Anthocyanins- Cyanidin
5. Biosynthesis of Phenyl Propanoids- Caffeic acid

Biosynthesis of Amino Acids

Amino acids are the precursors of some secondary metabolites particularly alkaloids. Plant synthesizes both the essential and non-essential amino acids. All amino acids are derived from intermediates in Glycolysis, the Citric acid cycle or the Pentose Phosphate Pathway. Fig.1.3 represents the overview of amino acid synthesis in plants.

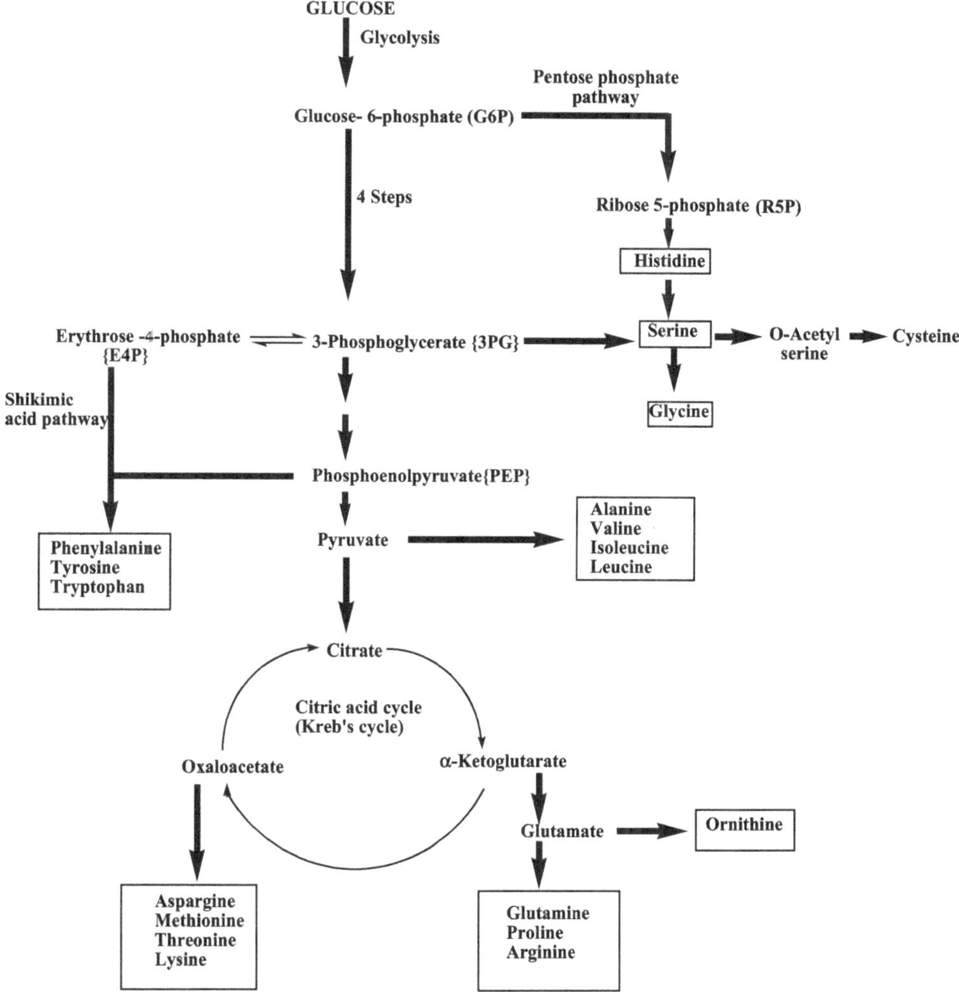

Fig. 1.3 Overview of Amino Acid synthesis

Biosynthesis of Phenylalanine, Tyrosine and Tryptophan (Aromatic amino acids)

The biosynthesis of Phenylalanine, Tyrosine and Tryptophan is well explained in Shikimic acid pathway.

Biosynthesis of Glutamate, Glutamine, Proline, Arginine and Ornithine

α- Ketoglutarate intermediate from Krebs cycle is involved in biosynthesis of several amino acids. The α-Ketoglutarate initially get converted into the amino acid glutamate in the presence of aminotransferase. This gutamate synthesizes the glutamine in presence of the enzyme glutamine synthetase. L-glutamate also involved in the synthesis of proline. Ornithine is a non-protein amino acid formed mainly from L-glutamate in plants and synthesized from the urea cycle. Arginine get synthesized through ornithine. The biosynthesis of proline, arginine is a complex biochemical chain of reactions. The possible biosynthesis can be represented as in figure1.3 (A).

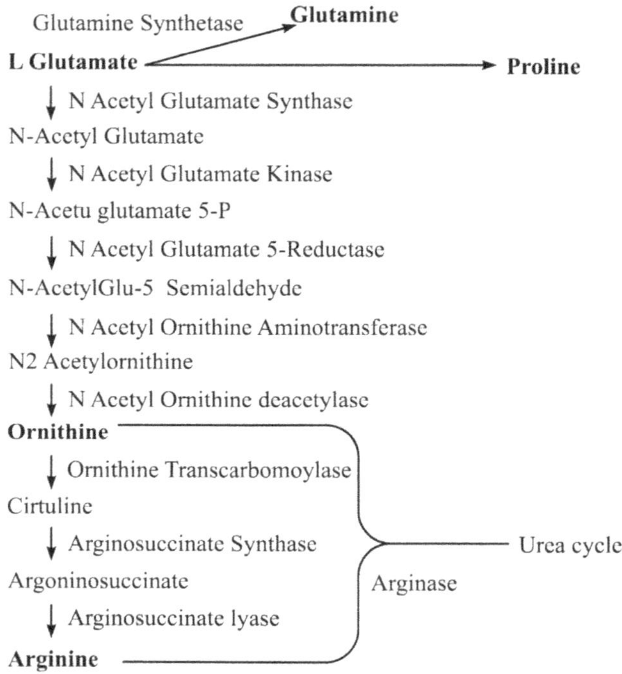

Fig. 1.3 (A) Overview of amino acid synthesis from L-Glutamate

Biosynthesis of Lysine, Aspargine, Methionine and Threonine

This is highly complex pathway which starts with intermediate of Kreb's cycle- Oxaloacetate. The oxaloacetate undergoes transamination to synthesize aspartate. In the presence of enzyme aspartokinase (catalyst) phsphorylation of aspartate takes place which initiates the conversion of aspartate to other amino acids. Lysine is synthesized from aspartate through diaminopimelate pathway. Aspartate also involves in biosynthesis of aspargine through aspargine synthetase enzyme. The intermediate aspartate 4-semialdehyde is produced which later involved in biosynthesis of methionine and threonine.

Biosynthesis of Serine, Glycine and Cysteine

Serine is the first amino acid produced from 3-phosphoglycerate which is originated from glycolysis through the enzyme phosphoglycerate dehydrogenase. The enzyme concentration in the cell is monitored by serine. Serine is then branched to synthesize other amino acids glycine and cysteine.

Biosyntheis of Alanine, Valine, Leucine and Isoleucine

Pyruvate is the key intermediate product of glycolysis which is involved in the biosynthesis of above amino acids. The few molecules of pyruvate is branched to synthesize alanine, valine, leucine and isoleucine and major part of pyruvate enters into Kreb's cycle.

Alanine is produced by the transamination of one molecule of pyruvate. Two molecules of pyruvates undergo condesation to produce α- acetolactic acid followed by α-keto-β-hydroxy valeric acid. The α-keto-β- hydroxy valeric acid is a intermediate to produce valine and leucine. It undergo reduction followed by transamination to synthesize valine. Similarly α-keto-β-hydroxy valeric acid undergoes acetate condensation and followed by sequence of reactions viz. reduction, dehydration and transamination to synthesize leucine

Isoleucine is produced by the same chain reaction as valine but starting with production of α-aceto-α-hydroxy propionic acid.

The Acetate – Mevalonate Pathway
(Mevalonic Acid Pathway/Isoprenoid Pathway)

The Acetate mevalonate pathway is also known as isoprenoid pathways as it results in the isoprenoid synthesis via formation of isoprene units. HMG-CoA reductase (3-hydroxy-3-methyl-glutaryl-CoA reductase) enzyme plays an important role in the formation of Mevalonic acid hence pathway also known as HMG-CoA pathway. Acetic acid plays an important role in the biosynthesis of cholesterol, squalene and many steroidal compounds which are synthesized through acetate pathway. In 1950's the discovery of acetyl Coenzyme A confirmed the role of acetic acid in biogenetic pathways.

Acetyl coenzyme A from citric acid cycle undergoes condensation with another molecule of acetyl coenzyme A to form Acetoacetyl CoA followed by condensation with another acetyl coenzyme A molecule to form 3-hydroxy-3-methyl-glutaryl-CoA (HMG-CoA). HMG-CoA get reduced to mevalonic acid. This Mevalonic acid acts as a precursor in the synthesis of isoprenoid compounds. The 'active isoprene' C_5 units; isopentenyl pyrophosphate (IPP) and its isomer dimethylallyl pyrophosphate (DMAPP) are the key intermediates synthesized by Mevalonic acid pathway. Both units yield Geranyl pyrophosphate (C_{10}- monoterpene). This Geranyl pyrophosphate again in association with IPP unit synthesizes Farnesyl pyrophosphate (C_{15} – sesquiterpene). Farnesyl pyrophosphate in further association with one IPP unit produces geranyl-geranyl pyrophosphate (C_{20} - diterpenes). This molecule further undergoes cyclization process to produce steroidal and penta cyclic triterpenoid skeleton. In this way acetate mevalonate pathway biosynthesizes wide range of monoterpenoids to pentacyclic triterpenoids.

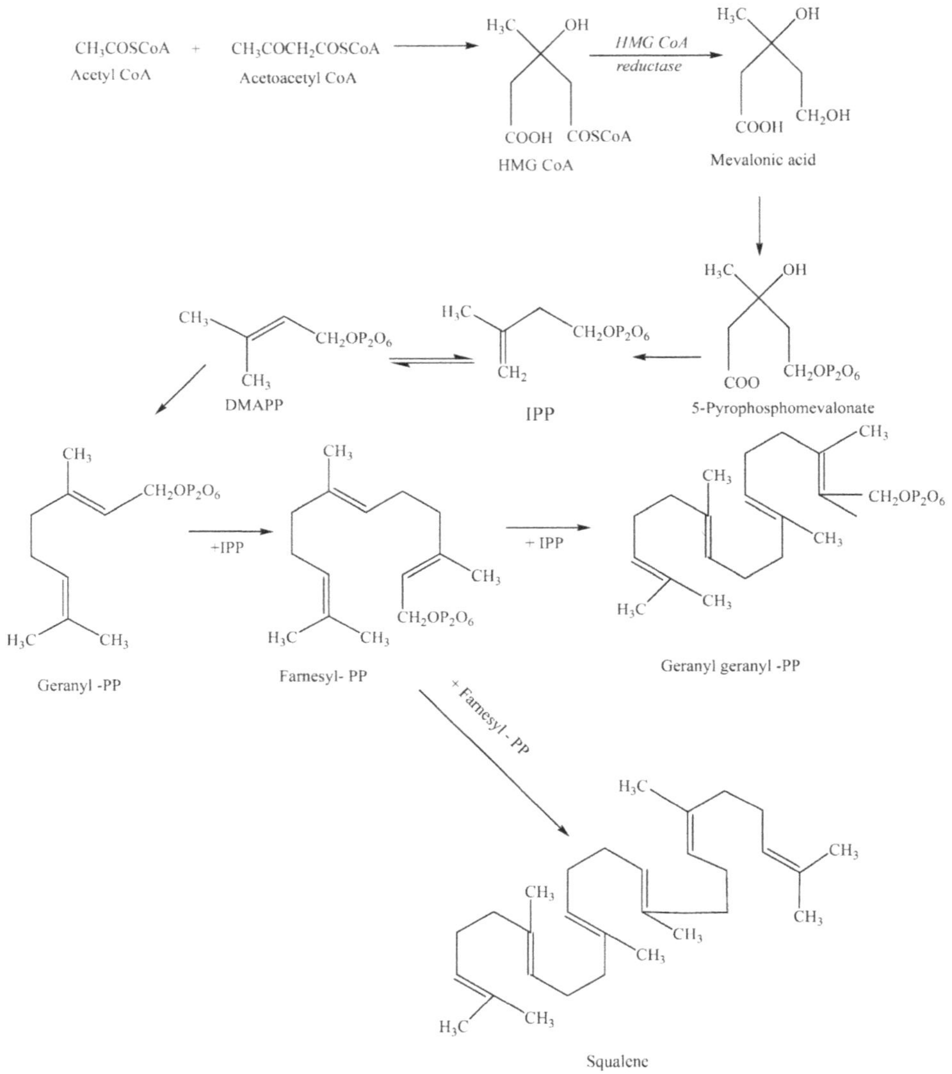

Fig. 1.4 The Acetate – Mevalonate Pathway

Acetate Malonate Pathway

The Acetate malonate pathway is mainly responsible for the synthesis of fatty acids which involves enzyme fatty acid synthase. It involves Acyl carrier protein (ACP) to yield fatty acid thioesters of ACP. These fatty acid thioesters form key intermediates in fatty acid synthesis. These C_2 acetyl CoA units further produce even number of fatty acids from butyric acid to arachidonic acid. Unsaturated acids are produced by subsequent direct dehydrogenation of saturated fatty acids. Enzymes involved in pathway plays an important role in governing position of newly introduced double bonds in the fatty acids.

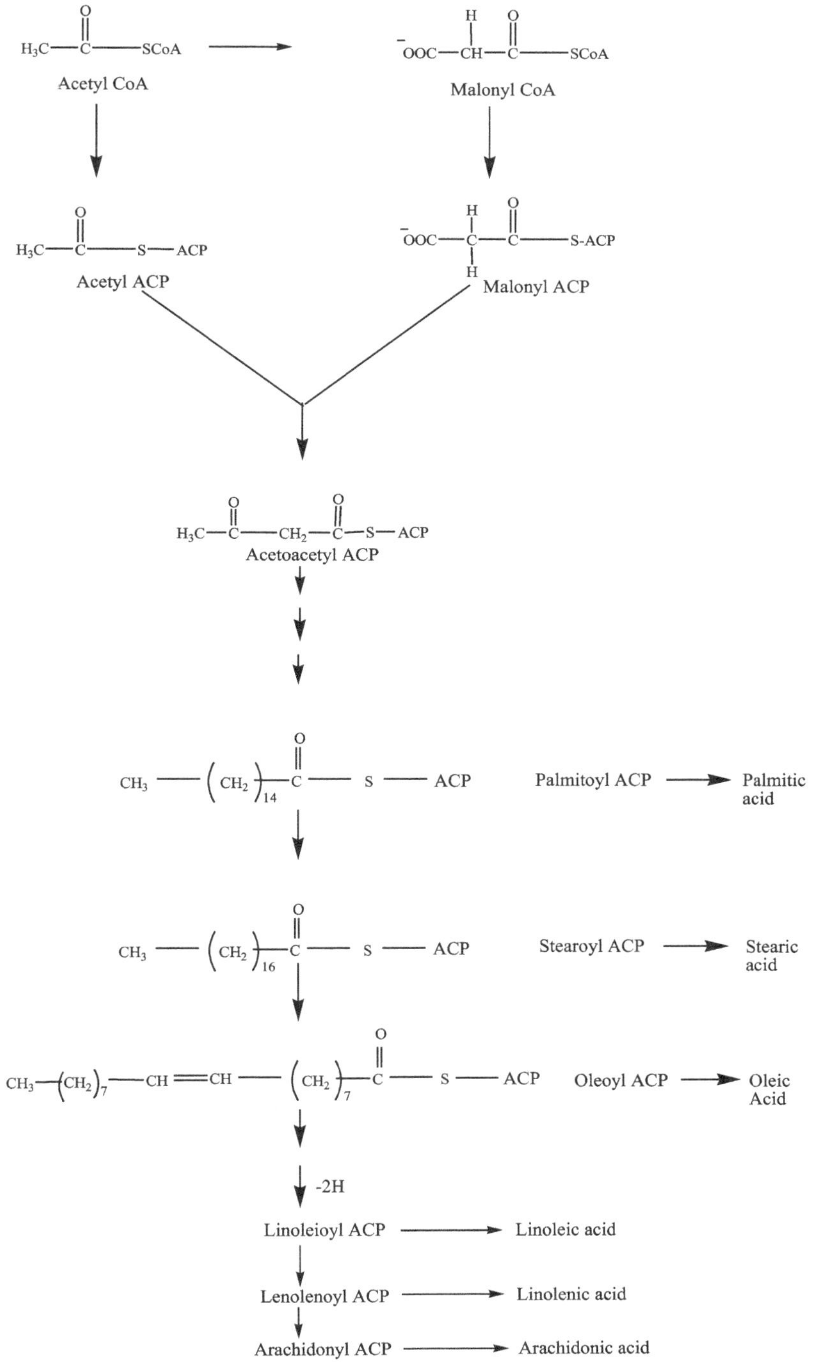

Acetyl CoA → Malonyl CoA

Acetyl ACP

Malonyl ACP

Acetoacetyl ACP

Palmitoyl ACP → Palmitic acid

Stearoyl ACP → Stearic acid

Oleoyl ACP → Oleic Acid

-2H

Linoleioyl ACP → Linoleic acid

Lenolenoyl ACP → Linolenic acid

Arachidonyl ACP → Arachidonic acid

Fig. 1.5 The Acetate Malonate Pathway

Biosynthesis of Secondary Metabolites

Biosynthesis of Glycosides

The glycosides are the condesation products of Glycone (sugar) and Aglycone (non sugar) units. The reaction occurs in two parts; the first part of biosynthesis is the formation of a aglycone part and second part is coupling of aglycone unit with glycone moity.

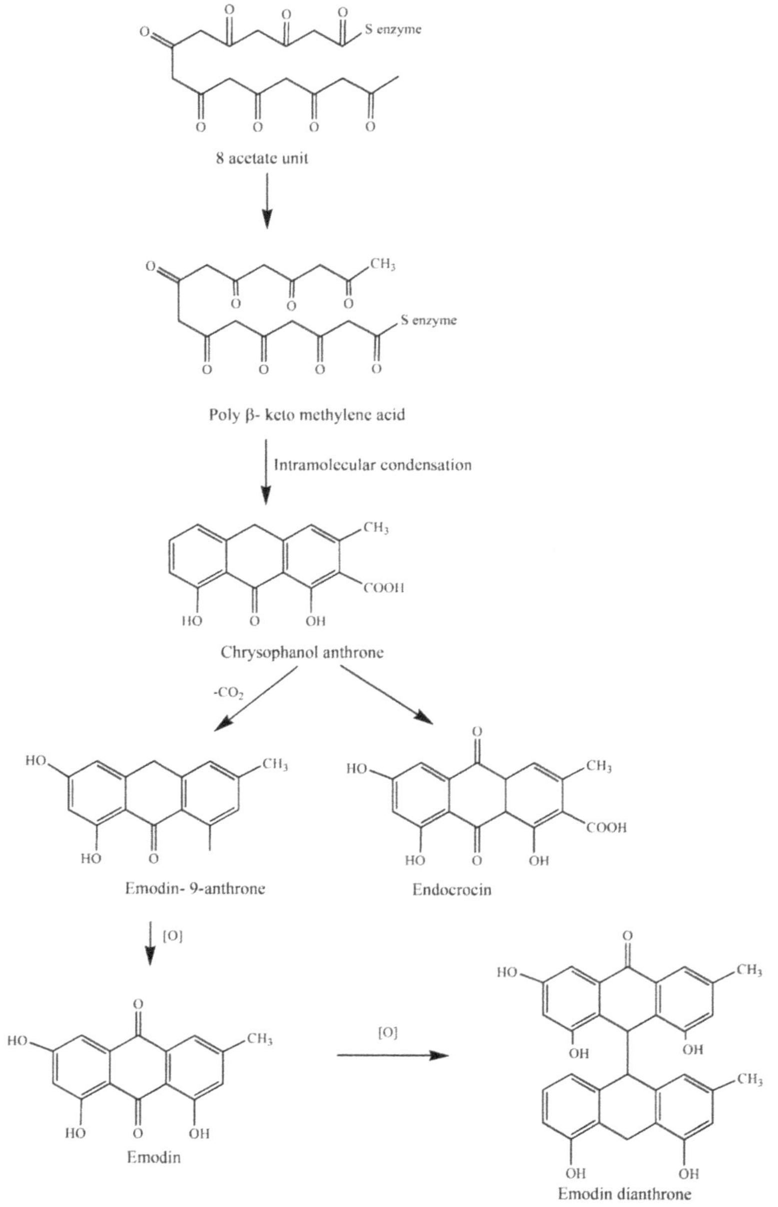

Fig. 1.6 Biosynthesis of Emodin and other Anthraquinone derivatives

The glycoside formation involves the transfer of uridyl group from uridine triphosphate (UTP) to sugar-1-phosphate in the presence of enzyme uridyl transferases to produce sugar-uridine diphosphate complex. In subsequent reaction this sugar nucleotide complex reacts with acceptor (Aglycone) units which leads to glycoside production.

$$\text{UTP + Sugar-1- phosphate} \underset{\text{Uridyl transferase}}{\rightleftharpoons} \text{UDP- Sugar + PP1}$$

$$\text{UDP- Sugar + Acceptor} \underset{\text{Glycosyl transferase}}{\rightleftharpoons} \text{Glycoside + UDP}$$

A. ***Biosynthesis of Anthracene Glycosides***: The knowledge of biosynthesis of anthracene aglycone has been established from the (Fig. 1.6) studies with microorganisms specifically *Penicillium islandicum.*

Synthesis of Emodin and other related derivatives: An intermediate poly β-ketomethylene acid is considered to be formed from 8-acetate unit which undergoes intermolecular condensation gives rise to emodin and other related anthraquinone derivatives.

Synthesis of Alizarin: The another pathway for production of anthraquinone glycoside is through the Shikimic acid – mevalonic acid mediators. This pathway can be observed in Rubiaceae family plants, eg: Biosynthesis of Alizarin from *Rubia tinctorum* (Rubiaceae).

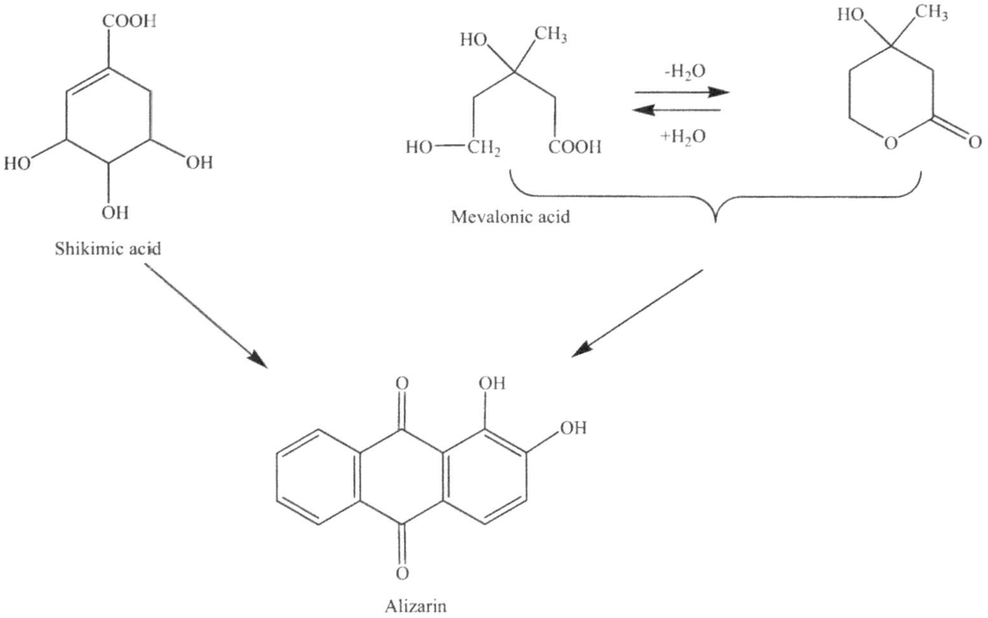

Fig. 1.7 Biosynthesis of Alizarin from *Rubia tinctorum* (Rubiaceae)

B. ***Biosynthesis of Cyanogenetic Glycosides***: The aglycone units of cyanogentic glycosides are the phenylpropanoid compounds derived from aromatic amino acids phenylalanine and tyrosine obtained from Shikimic acid pathway, eg; Prunacin and Dhurrin.

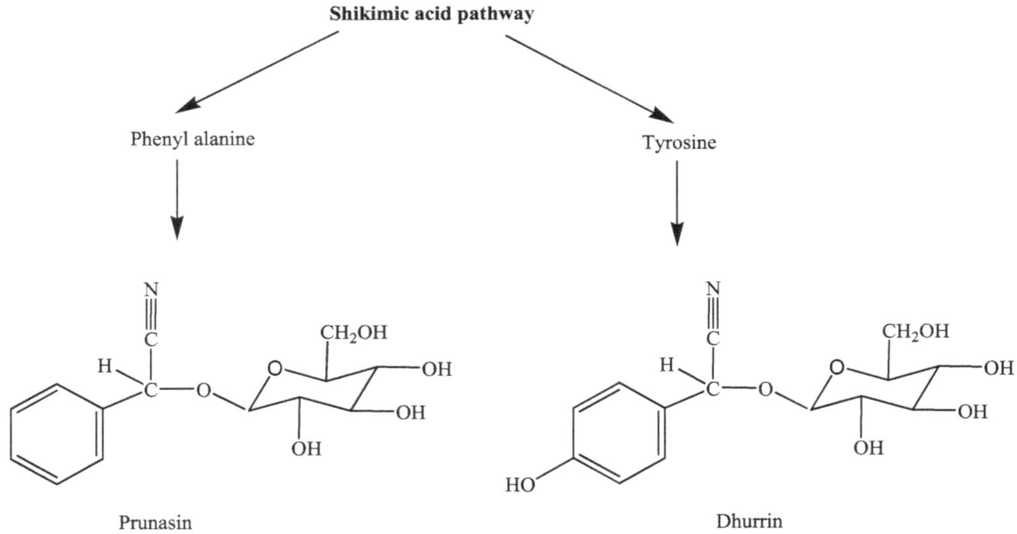

Fig. 1.8 Biosynthesis of Cyanogenetic Glycosides

C. *Biosynthesis of Isothiocyanate aglycone*: The aglycones of isothiocyanate may consist of either aliphatic derivative biosynthesized via acetate pathway or aromatic derivatives produced biosynthetically via Shikimic acid route.

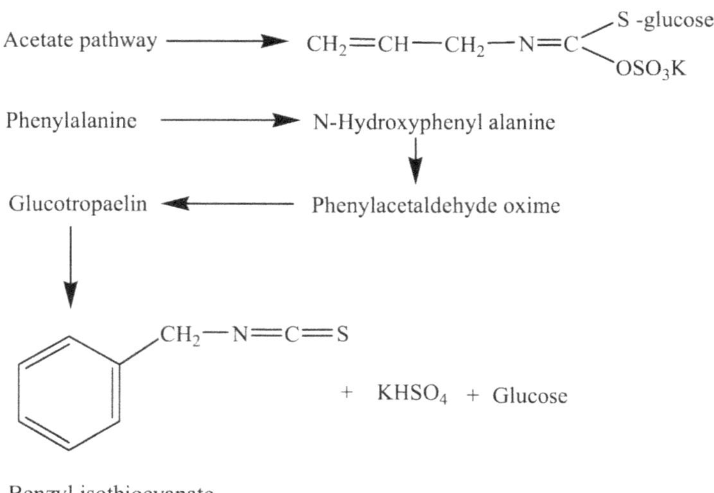

Fig. 1.9 Biosynthesis of Isothiocyanate Aglycone

D. *Biosynthesis of Flavonoid Aglycone*: The aglycones of Flavonol glycosides are derived from both acetate metabolism and Shikimic acid athway. The A ring arises by head –to-tail condensation of two malonyl Co-A units and Acetyl Co-A unit. The B ring and C_3 unit comes from a C_6-C_3 precursor, which may be cinnamic acid.

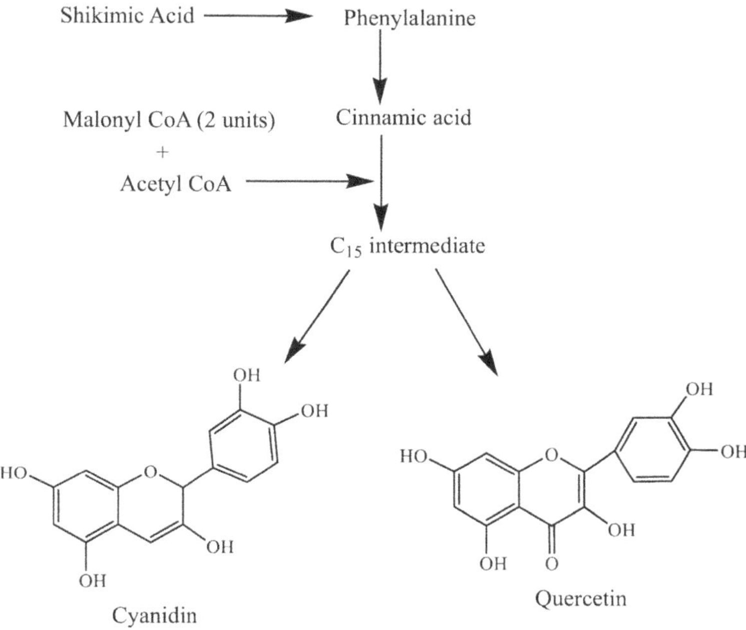

Fig. 1.10 Biosynthesis of Flavonoid Aglycone

E. ***Biosynthesis of Lactone, Phenol, Alcohol and aldehyde Glycoside***: The aromatic nuclei of alcohol, aldehyde, lactone and phenol glycosides are derived from C_6-C_3 precursor formed via Shikimc acid pathway.

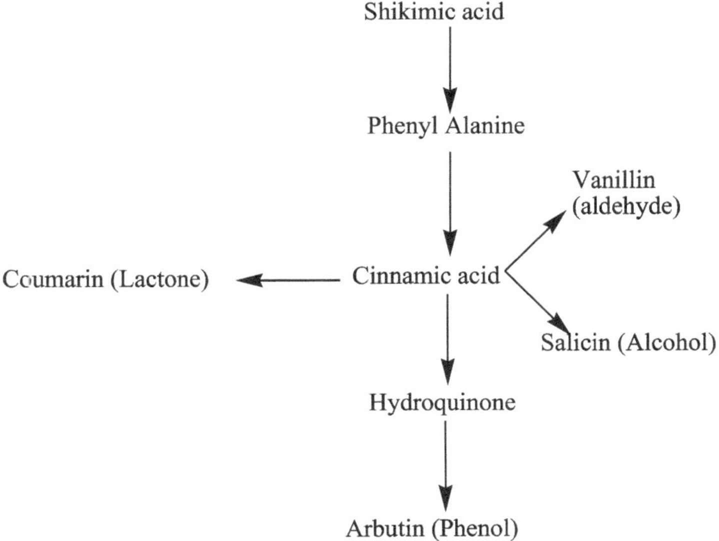

Fig. 1.11 Biosynthesis of Lactone, Phenol, Alcohol and aldehyde Glycoside

F. Biosynthesis of Aglycones of Cardiac Glycosides and Saponins: The aglycones of cardio active glycosides are steroidal in nature. They are the derivatives of cyclopentanophenanthrene ring which contains the following.

An unsaturated lactone ring attached to C 17 ,

A 14-α Hydroxyl group and

A cis- juncture of rings C & D

The steroidal biosynthesis is relatively similar to the cholesterol production via Acetate, Mevalonate, isopentenyl pyrophosphate followed by squaline pathway. The biosynthesis of cholesterol involves cyclization of aliphatic triterpene-squalene. Eg: Biosynthesis of Digitoxigenin, Digoxigenin and Gitoxigenin.

Similarly neutral sapogenins (saponin glycosides) are derivatives of steroids while acid sapogenins possess triterpenoids. Both the sapogenins are biosynthesized by similar pathway till the production of triterpenoid hydrocarbon squalene. This further branches to give cyclic triterpenoid in one direction and steroids in another direction. Figure 1.12 shows the brief outline of biosynthesis of certain steroidal compounds viz. squalene, cholesterol, digitoxigenin, scillarennin etc.

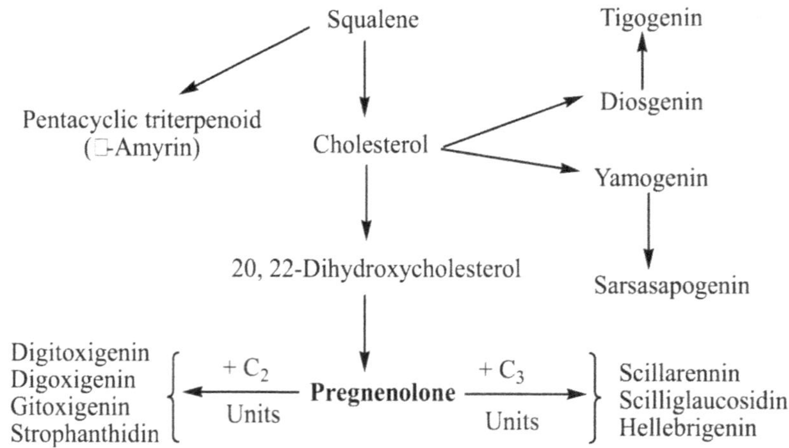

Fig. 1.12 Biosynthesis of steroidal aglycone

Biosynthesis of Alkaloids

Alkaloids are the nitrogen containing compounds; some derived from purines / pyrimidines and majority are produced from amino acids. Ornithine produces pyrrolidine and tropane alkaloids while lysine gives piperidine, quinolizidine, and indolizidine alkaloids. Similarly, nicotinic acid gives rise to pyridine alkaloids and tyrosine produces phenyl ethylamines and simple tetra hydroisoquinoline alkaloids. Pharmacologically important alkaloids are discussed below;

A. *Alkaloids derived from ornithine*: Ornithine is a precursor of the cyclic pyrrolidines *viz.* alkaloids of tobacco (nicotine, nornicotine) and other plants of Solanaceae family. The amino acid ornithine on decarboxylation produces putrescine and proline- the basic unit of tropane, ecgonine and nicotine group of alkaloids (pyrolidine ring).

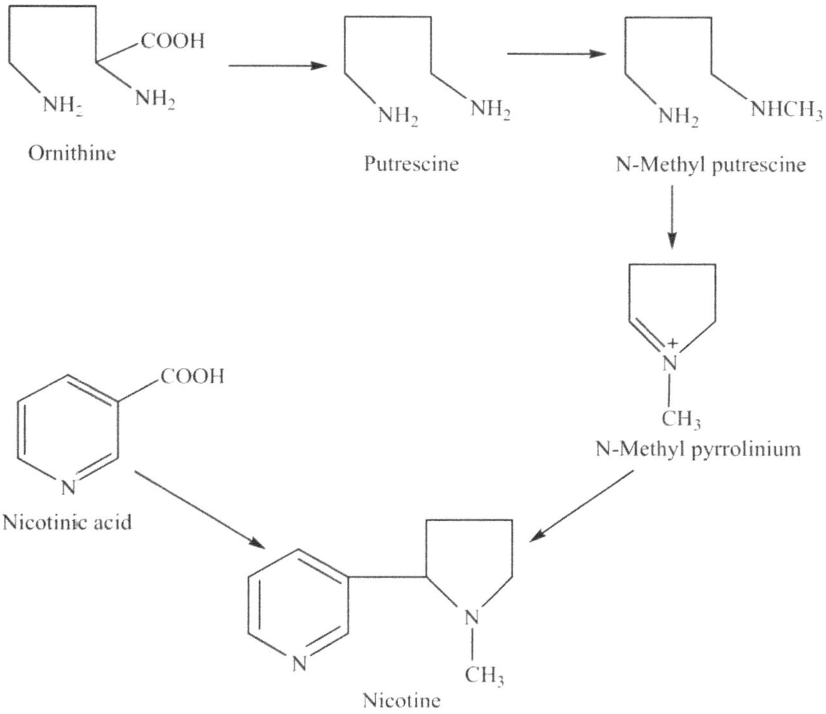

Fig. 1.13 Biosynthesis of Nicotine

B. *Alkaloids derived from lysine*: Lysine is a precursor for piperidine which forms the basic skeleton for many alkaloids. Lysine and its derivatives are responsible for the biosynthesis of some of the bitter principles *viz.* lupine, lupanine, anabasine and other related compounds.

$$3\text{L-lysine} \longrightarrow 3\text{-cadaverine} \longrightarrow 17\text{-oxosparteine} \longrightarrow \text{lupanine}$$

Fig. 1.14 Biosynthesis of Lupanine

C. *Alkaloids derived from phenyl alanine, tyrosine and related amino acids*: The amino acids phenyl alanine, tyrosine and related amino acids and their respective decarboxylation products serve as a precursor for many alkaloids. Tyrosine is considered to be a precursor for the huge family containing alkaloids. The first essential intermediate is dopamine; dopamine is the precursor in the biosynthesis of papaverine, berberine, and morphine.

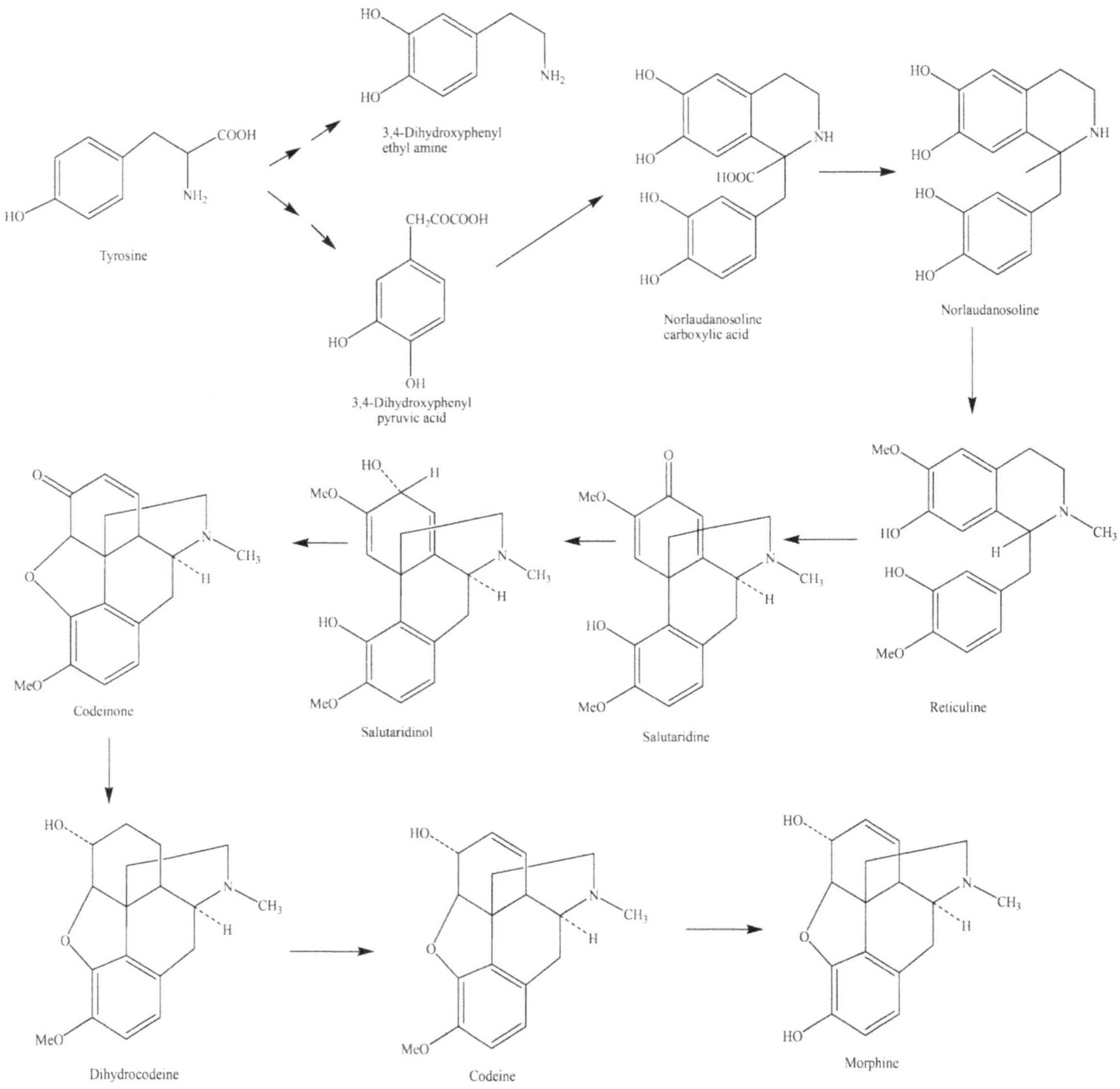

Fig. 1.15 Biosynthesis of Morphine

D. Alkaloids derived from tryptophan: Important group of alkaloid derived from tryptophan is indole alkaloids. Tryptophan and its decarboxylation product tryptamine, serve as a precursor for biosynthesis of a large number of indole alkloids. The biosynthesis of quinine and related alkaloids in cinchona takes place through the tranformation of indole to quinine.

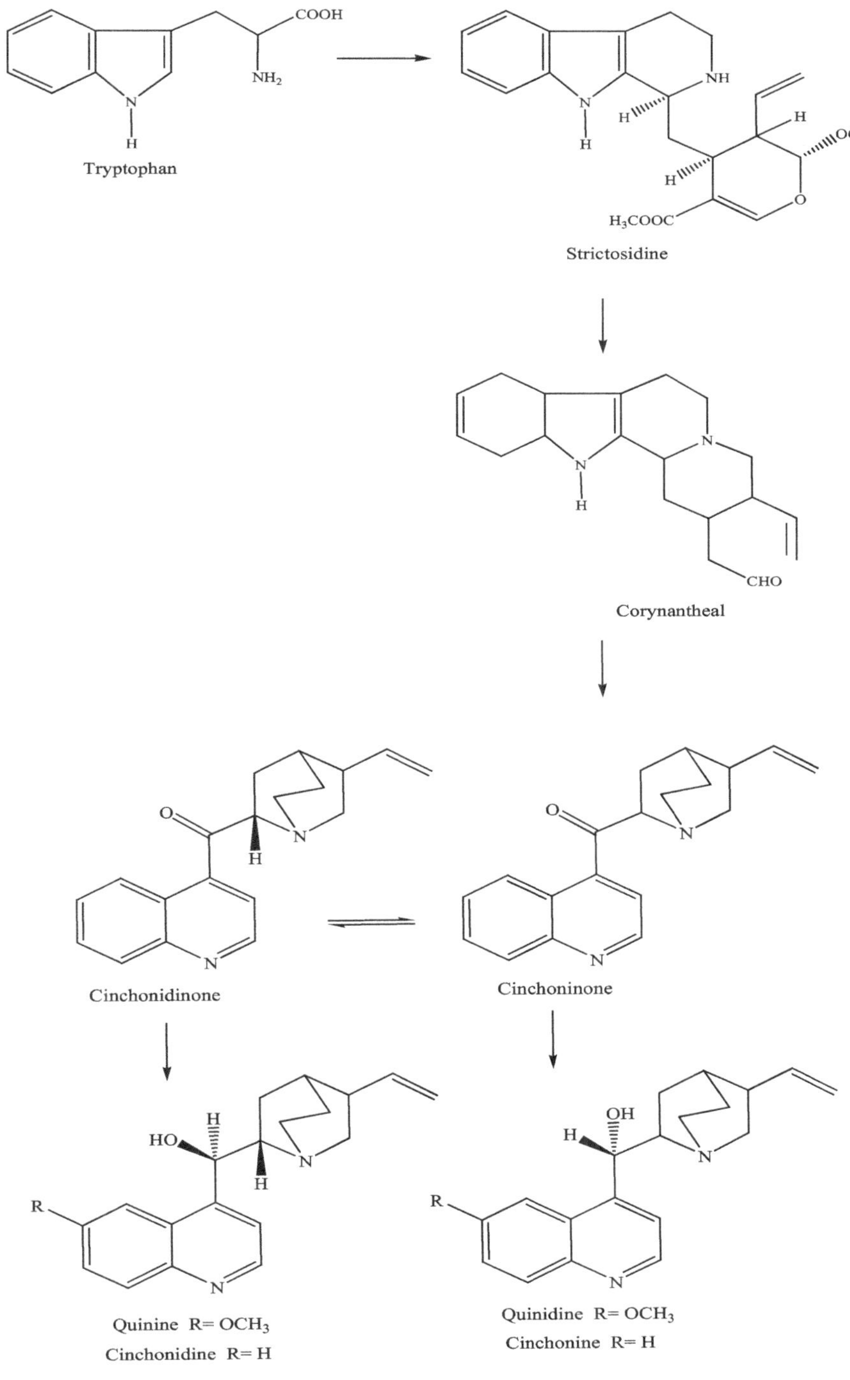

Fig 1.16 Biosynthesis of Cinchona alkaloids

Biosynthesis of Isoprenoid Compounds

Polymeric isoprene derivatives viz. steroids, carotenoids, gibberellic acid etc. though shows structural variation, are synthesized by very few pathways. To understand the biosynthesis of isoprenoid compound, acetate mevalonate pathway can be reffered.

Biosynthesis of Triglycerides (Fats and Fatty Acids)

Biosynthesis of triglycerides occurs in two stages; biosynthesis of fatty acid and formation of triglyceride. (Refer Acetate malonate pathway).

Biosynthesis of Phenolic Compounds

Most of the phenolic compounds are flavonoids. Flavonoids have basic skeleton from C_{15} body of flavones. Flavones occures both as colored and colorless nature. Some of the common phenolic compounds are coumarin, flavone, flavonol, anthocyanidines.

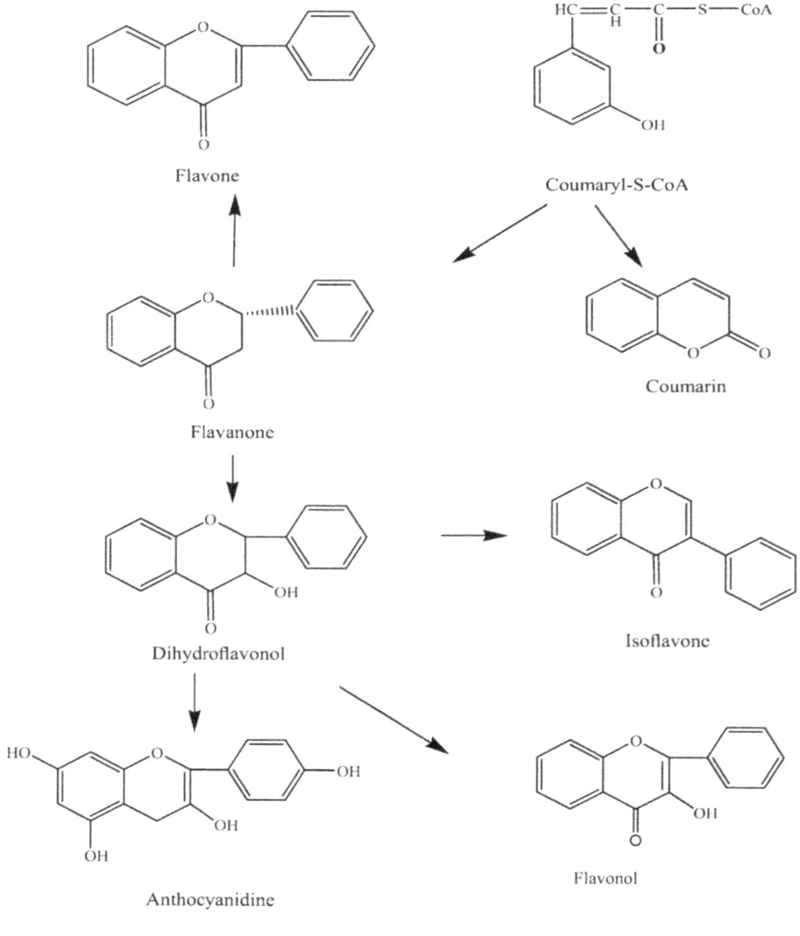

Fig. 1.17 Biosynthesis of Phenolic Compounds

Stress Compounds

These are the compounds which accumulate in the plants at higher than a normal level as a result of the biotic stress (attack by the pathogens, insects or herbivores) or abiotic stress (particularly contamination by heavy metals and different types of fertilizers) or due to injury or disturbances in normal metabolism (due to polymerization, oxidation or hydrolysis of natural substances). These are the products of primary or secondary metabolism. Several environmental and biological factors promote the synthesis of stress compounds these include mechanical wounding of plants, salinization, frost damage, desertification, drought, exposure to cold and salt. Chemically stress compounds are of different nature which includes phenols, resins, carbohydrates, hydroxycinnamic acid derivatives, coumarins, bicyclic sesquiterpenes, triterpenes and steroidal compounds. Stress compounds are also of pharmaceutical importance as they may be involved in various crude drugs formed pathologically *viz.* gums and oleoresins are potential drugs. Phytoalexins is one of the examples of stress compounds produced as an antifungal by plants after fungal infestation. The antifungal isoflavonoid pterocarpans produced by many species of Leguminosae family as a stress compound.

Study of Utilization of Radioactive Isotopes in the Investigation of Biogenetic Studies

Investigation of biogenetic pathways are generally carried out by using the radioactive isotopes.

Isotopes: Isotopes of a given element have nuclei with the same number of protons but different numbers of neutrons. They have different physical properties but the same chemical properties. Some isotopes are stable; however, radioisotopes are unstable and disintegrate, with the emission of three main types of radiation- alpha, beta and gamma radiations. A radioisotope, or any compound that contains a radioisotope, is said to be radiolabeled and is called a radionuclide. Each radioisotope has a characteristic rate of decay and pattern of radiation. For example, 14-C is a low energy beta emitter with a half-life of 5500 years. The labelled compounds are prepared using radioactive isotopes. The common radioactive isotopes in wide use are ^{14}C, ^{3}H, ^{35}S, ^{32}P, ^{36}Cl, ^{131}I, ^{60}Co. Different isotopes are used in different studies; nitrogen atom is used in the studies on proteins, alkaloids and amino acids; carbon and hydrogen are useful in biological investigations and metabolic pathways and oxygen is useful in studies on terpenoids.

Many methods have been used for the investigation of different metabolic pathways by using radiolabeled compounds and they are as follows

Tracer Techniques

Tracer techniques are the techniques which utilizes a labelled radioactive compound/ isotope to find out the different intermediates and various steps involved in biosynthetic pathways in a plant at a given time and rate. These compounds after administration in the plant become a part of general metabolic pathway of the plant and undergo characteristic metabolic reactions associated with plant metabolism. The different types of tracer techniques are as follows.

- Use of isolated organs

- Grafting methods

- Use of mutant strain

Criteria for selection of tracer

- The physical and chemical nature of the presumed precursor of biochemical reaction must be known for proper labeling.

- The initial concentration of labeled compound must be sufficient to complete the targeted biogenetic pathway.

- The labeled isotope should be of a sufficiently longer half-life.

- The labeled compound should not damage the system into which it has been inserted.

Steps involved in tracer techniques

1. Preparation of radio labeled compound.

2. Introduction of labeled compound into a biological system.

3. Separation of the labeled compound and determination of nature of metabolites in various biochemical fractions.

1. **Preparation of radio labeled compound:** The different radioactive isotopes are prepared by different methods. The radioactive ^{14}C can be prepared synthetically and naturally. The purity of ^{14}C used for biochemical investigations is highly important. ^{14}C can be prepared by two methods;

   A. By the bombardment of ^{14}N with slow neutrons on the target material viz aluminum beryllium nitride in nuclear reactor. The disadvantage is that the labeled carbon produced by this method may contaminate with inorganic radioactive carbon compounds.

   B. The other method used is by growing algae *Chlorella* in an atmosphere containing $^{14}CO_2$. All the carbon compounds of the organism thus become labeled, possessing uniform labeling of each carbon atom.

   Tritium ^{3}H is effected by catalytic exchange (Platinum catalyst) in aqueous media, by irradiation of organic compounds with tritium gas and by hydrogenation of unsaturated compounds with tritium gas.

2. **Introduction of labeled compound into a biological system**

   Before the selection of method for introduction of radiolabeled compounds, the following precautions must be taken

   - The presumed precursor should introduce at specific site so that it takes part in the biochemical reaction.

   - The introduction time of labeled compound should be correct so that the presumed precursor should be available during the biosynthesis of the compound.

- The dose should be as minimum as possible to avoid the involvement of labeled compound in other biochemical reactions

The different methods for introduction of labeled compounds are available. These are:

Root feeding: The plants in which the roots are site for biosynthetic reactions for production of targeted compounds, root feeding technique is used. e.g. Production of Datura and tobacco alkaloids. The plants are hydroponically cultivated to avoid microbial contamination along with labeled compound.

Stem feeding: Substrate can be administered through cut ends of stem immersed in solution with necessary nutrients and labeled compounds. The stems which oozes latex after cutting are not suitable for this method.

Direct injection: This is the easiest method for introduction of labeled compounds. Direct injection is possible for those plants which bears the hollow stems. e.g. Opium

Infiltration: This method is suitable for the plants rooted in soil or with other support. The infiltration method enables to introduce the labeled compounds without disturbing the roots (wick feeding).

Floating methods: This method is used when small amount of material is available. This technique is used in conjugation with vacuum infiltration to remove gases.

Spray technique: The radiolabeled compound is mixed in water and then spread over the leaves. The compound gets absorbed in the leaves and participate in metabolic pathways. e.g steroids.

3. **Separation of the labeled compound and determination of nature of metabolites in various biochemical fractions**

Separation of labeled compounds: For the successful separation of radiolabeled compound from the part of plants, different methods and solvents are used based on the nature of the part of the plant. For soft and fresh tissue maceration or infusion is used. For hard tissue decoction or percolation is used and for separation of labeled compound from unorganized drug maceration with adjustments is preferred.

Depending upon the nature of the presumed product, the solvent is selected for separation *viz.* for fats and oils, nonpolar solvents are used while for alkaloids, glycosides slightly polar solvents are used and for phenols polar solvents are used.

Determination of labeled compounds: The different types of detectors are used for identification of radiolabeled compounds as mentioned below.

- Geiger – Muller counter
- Scintillators
- Autoradiography
- Mass spectroscopy
- NMR spectroscopy
- Gas ionization chamber

- Bernstein – Bellentine counter
- Radio paper chromatography

Important methods of determination of radiolabeled compounds are explained here.

Geiger – Muller Counter

The Geiger – Muller (GM) counter is an instrument used for measuring the ionizing radiation. It detects ionizing radiations *viz.* alpha particles, beta particles and gamma radiations using the ionization effect produced in a Geiger – Muller tube. A Geiger counter consists of a Geiger Muller tube with pair of electrodes, the sensing element which detects the radiation, processing units and results in display. Geiger Muller tube is filled with an inert gas such as helium, neon, or argon at low pressure and to this high voltage is applied. When radiation enters the tube, it ionizes the gas, the ions get attracted towards the electrode and an electric current is produced. A scale counts the current pulses and one can get the count whenever radiations ionizes the gas.

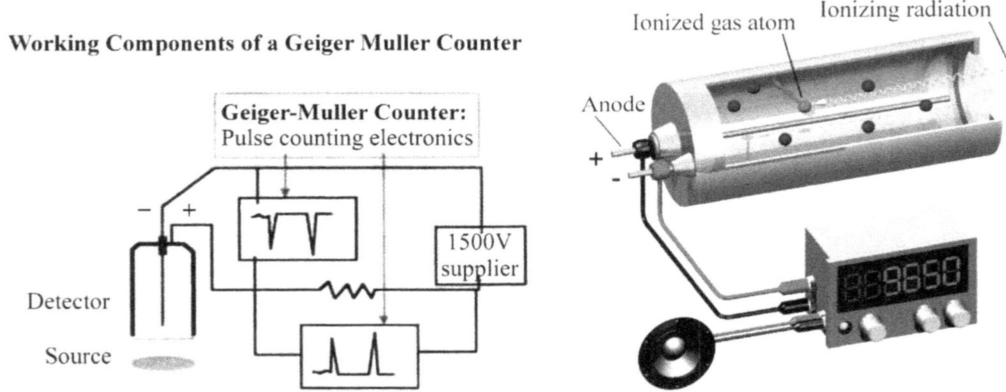

Fig. 1.18 Components of Geiger Muller counter

Advantages: It is relatively economical, durable, easily portable and detects all types of radiations.

Disadvantages: It cannot differentiate the type of radiation is being detected. It has less sensitivity and efficacy.

Scintillators

Scintillations literal meaning is luminescence and scintillators are materials which have property of luminescence, when excited by ionizing radiation. Scintillation counter is an instrument for detecting and measuring the ionizing radiations by using the excitation effect of incident radiation on a scintillator material and detecting the resultant light pulses. The scintillators detect the radiation with the help of photomultiplier tube that gives rise to an equivalent electric pulse. When an ionizing particle passes into the scintillator material, atoms are ionized along a track. The photon from the scintillation strikes a photocathode and emits an electron which accelerated by a pulse and produce a voltage across the external resistance. This voltage is amplified and recorded by an electron counter.

Applications: Scintillator counters are used to measure radiation in a variety of applications including handheld radiations survey meters, personal and environmental monitoring for radioactive contamination, medical imaging, radiometric assay, nuclear security, and nuclear plant safety.

Advantages: It can accommodate samples of any type including liquids, solids, suspensions and gels.

* Easy sample preparation methods.

* It can count separately different isotopes in the same sample so dual labeling experiments can be carried out.

* Scintillators are highly automated, efficient and highly accurate.

Disadvantages:

* It is very expensive.

* If high voltage applied to photomultiplier, electronic events occurs in the system that are independent of radioactivity known as photomultiplier noise.

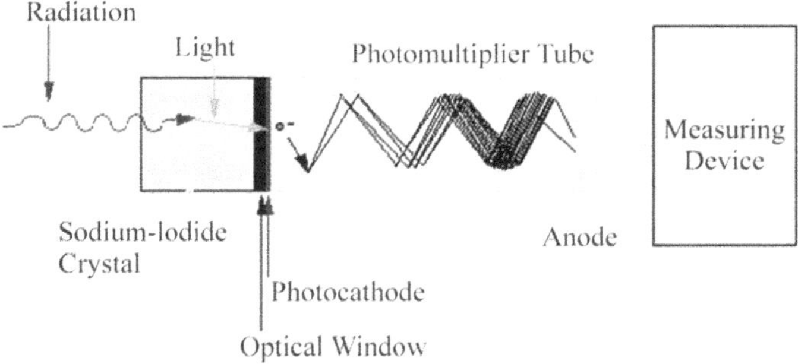

Fig 1.19 The photomultiplier Scintillator

Autoradiography

Autoradiography is the bio-analytical technique used to visualize the distribution of radioactive labeled substance with radioisotope in a biological sample. It is a method by which a radioactive material can be localized within a particular tissue, cell, cell organelles or even biomolecules. Autoradiography is based upon the ability of radioactive substance to expose the photographic film by ionizing it. In this technique a radioactive substance is put into direct contact with a thick layer of a photographic emulsion (thickness of 5-50 mm) having gelatin substances and silver halide crystals. It is then left in dark for several days for proper exposure. The silver halide crystals are exposed to the radiation which chemically converts silver halide into metallic silver (reduced) giving a dark color band. The resulting radiography is viewed by electron microscope, preflashed screen, intensifying screen, electrophoresis or digital scanners. It is a very sensitive technique and is being used in a wide variety of biological experiments. Autoradiography, although used to locate the radioactive substances, it can also be used for quantitative estimation by using densitometer.

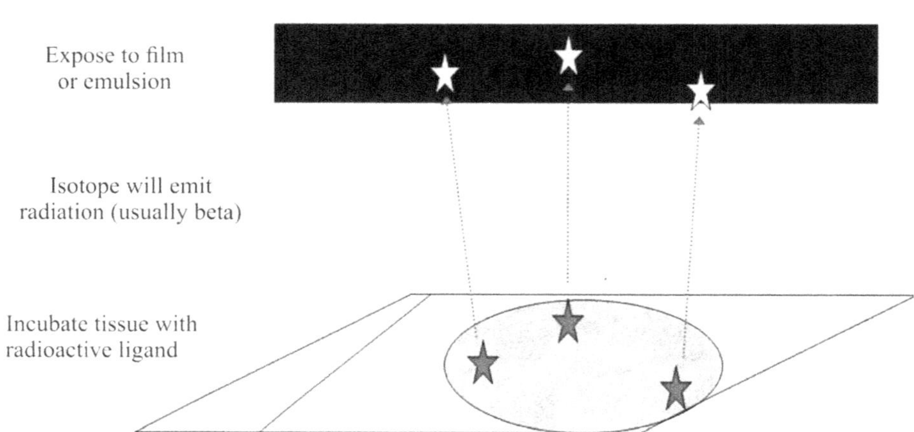

Fig. 1.20 Autoradiography

Applications

- To find and investigate the various properties of DNA.
- To find the location and amount of particular substance within a cell including cell organelle, metabolites etc.
- Tissue localization of radioactive substance.
- To find out the site and performance of targeted drug.
- To locate the metabolic activity site in the cell.

Mass Spectrophotometer

Mass spectrometry (MS) is an analytical technique that measures the mass-to-charge ratio of charged particles. It is used for determining masses of particles, for determining the elemental composition of a sample or molecule, and for elucidating the chemical structures of molecules, such as peptides and other chemical compounds.

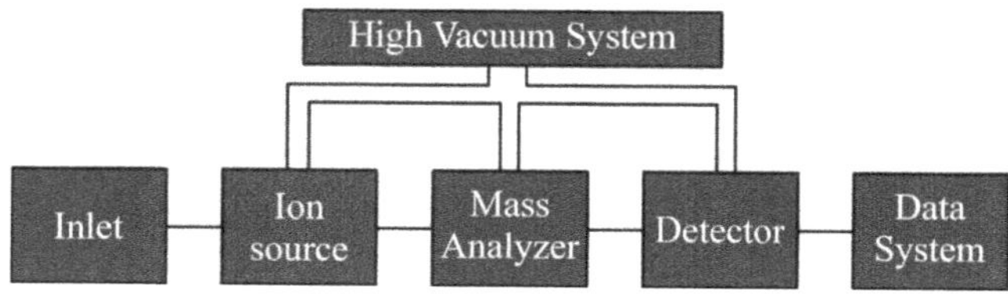

Fig 1.21 Block diagram of Mass Spectrophotometer

NMR Spectrophotometer

NMR spectroscopy is an analytical technique that measures the magnetic properties of certain atomic nuclei to determine physical and chemical properties of atoms or the molecules. It relies on the phenomenon of nuclear magnetic resonance and can provide detailed information about the structure, dynamics, reaction state, and chemical environment of molecules.

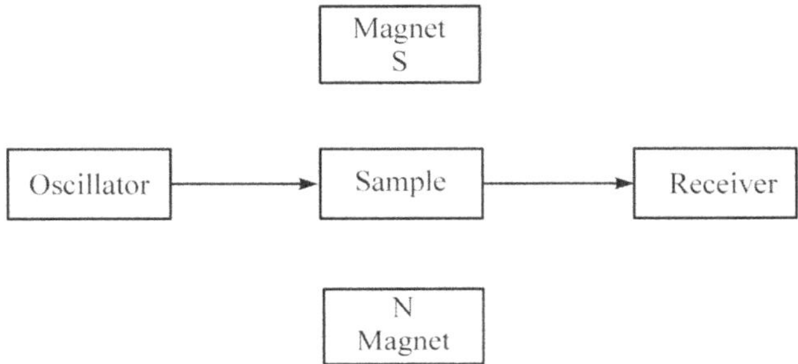

Fig. 1.22 Simple block diagram of NMR spectrophotometer

Other Techniques to Investigate Biosynthetic Pathways

Precursor Product Sequence

This is the most used technique for the elucidation of biosynthetic pathways in plants by using labeled compounds. In this technique, a presumed precursor of the constituent under investigation on a labeled form is fed into the plant and after a suitable time the constituent is isolated, purified and radioactivity is determined. Generally, the radioactivity of the isolated compound is not sufficient evidence to confirm the precursor –product sequence because labeled compound may enter the general metabolic pathways of the plants and from there may get randomly distributed through a whole range of biochemical reactions. If this happens degradation of isolated compound and determination of the activity of the fragment may not be able to give specific precursor product sequence. Therefore, for investigation of correct precursor product sequence, double or triple labeling either of different isotopes or specific labeling by one isotope at two or more positions in the molecule is employed. The double-triple labeling is widely used technique for the investigation of secondary metabolites in the plants. e.g. The best experimental example is incorporation of doubly labeled lysine into anabasine. It is known that lysine is precursor for anabasine. The double labeled lysine for the investigation of biogenesis of anabasine confirms which nitrogen of lysine molecule is involved in formation of pyridine ring of anabasine in *Nicotiana glauca*. In the experiment lysine labeled with C_2-^{15}N and C_6-^{15}N introduced, in the final product C_6-^{15}N retained instead of C_2-^{15}N.

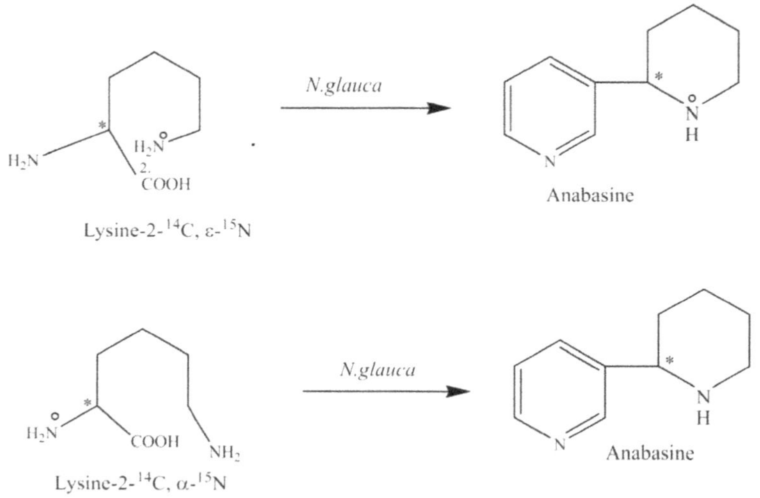

Lysine-2-^{14}C, ε-^{15}N → (N.glauca) → Anabasine

Lysine-2-^{14}C, α-^{15}N → (N.glauca) → Anabasine

Fig. 1.23 Incorporation of doubly labeled lysine into anabasine

Applications

- Stopping of hordenine production in barley seedling after days of germination.
- Restricted synthesis of hyoscine, distinct from hyoscyamine in *Datura stramonium.*
- This method is applied to the biogenesis of Morphine & Ergot alkaloids.

Competitive Feeding

In this technique, the labeled compounds used to determine precursor and exact intermediates. In plants, the biosynthesis of phytoconstituents is a very complex process which involves the many possibilities / probabilities for their precursors and intermediates and final products. It is always difficult and confusing task to predict them. Competitive feeding technique has great value in distinguishing the normal intermediate in the formation of phytoconstituents. The given example can explain the role of competitive feeding technique in identifying the intermediates.

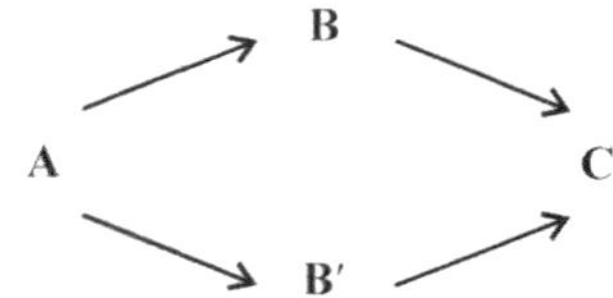

Fig. 1.24 Competitive feeding

In figure 1.24, A is the precursor and C is end product which synthesized through either B or B' as intermediates. The plant fed with labeled A act as control. Two other plants are fed with radiolabeled A simultaneously with radioactive B' in one plant and inactive B in another plant. If the incorporation or presence of labeled compounds into C is inhibited in the plants receiving B but is unaffected in the plant receiving B'; then we may confirm that the pathway from A to C proceeds via B.

Applications

- This method is used for elucidation of biogenesis of tropane alkaloids.

Sequential Analysis

This is another simple method for investigation of biogenetic pathways by using $^{14}CO_2$. In this technique, plant is grown in an atmosphere of $^{14}CO_2$ and plant parts are subjected to analysis at given time interval. This analysis provides the information about the sequence in which the various compounds become labeled. Most of the biosynthetic pathways are lengthy and complex, from the results of analysis certain biosynthetic pathways can be confirmed and some can be rejected.

This method has been very successfully implemented in the elucidation of the path of carbon in photosynthesis and also in the determination of sequential formation of alkaloids from opium, hemlock and tobacco. In one experiment very short period of 5 minutes exposure to $^{14}CO_2$ is used to investigate the biosynthetic sequence piperitone, menthone, menthol in *Mentha piperita*.

Use of Stable Isotopes

The stable isotopes ^{2}H, ^{13}C, ^{15}N and ^{18}O, which have a low natural occurrence can be used in similar way as radioactive elements for labeling compounds to be used as possible intermediates in biosynthetic pathways. The intermediate analysis can be done by using techniques like Mass spectroscopy and NMR spectroscopy.

Use of Isolated Organs Tissues or Cells

The cultivation of isolated organs, tissues and cells in suitable media is one of the techniques to investigate the biosynthetic pathway. It eliminates interference from other parts of the plant which may produce secondary changes in the metabolites. It is useful for the determination of the site of synthesis of particular compounds. Furthermore, it facilitates the easy introduction of labeled compound to parenchyma cells of tissue organ such as shoots, roots, petals, leaves etc.

Isolated part of the plants when placed in suitable solution or water, will have normal metabolism after separation from the plant this is the basis of this method. The isolated parts are grown on sterile nutrient media in aseptic condition. The radiolabeled compounds are added to the culture to study the biogenetic pathway. This method has the advantage that the nutrient solution or water medium does not requires sugar as sufficient starch is synthesized in the leaf and consequently bacterial and fungal growth in the nutrient solution is minimized. The isolated shoot end is placed in suitable nutrient media containing radiolabeled compound while isolated roots/ leaves are dipped in the media containing radiolabeled compounds. By using this technique tropane alkaloid are produced in the roots of Solanaceae family plants and number of precursors are incorporated to investigate the biogenetic pathway of alkaloids.

Use of Grafts

Grafting technique is particularly used for the determination of the sites of primary and secondary metabolism in plants. Grafting is an art of joining two different plant parts together in such a manner that they unite and continue their growth as a single plant. The upper portion of the one plant (stem/bud) known as scion is joined with stock/rootstock (stem/root/branch) of another plant in such a way that their tissue joined together to grow further.

Alkaloid formation by grafted plants has been studied extensively in Nicotiana and Datura. In this method tomato scions grafted onto Datura stocks accumulate tropane alkaloids whereas Datura scions on tomato stocks contain only small amount of tropane alkaloids. This indicates that site of alkaloids biosynthesis is Datura roots.

Grafting has its own limitations viz., grafting is possible only in dicots, possible between two different genera in the same family, and possible between two different species in the same genus. There are several techniques available for grafting; Scion attached method (inarching, saddle grafting or tongue grafting), Scion detached methods (veneer grafting, wedge grafting, whip and tongue grafting, softwood grafting), methods of grafting on established trees (side grafting, crown grafting) and methods of renovation (bridge grafting).

Use of Mutant Strains

Mutant strains are the species which are produced due to change in genetic characters. This results in the physical and physiological changes. Either physical methods (through radiation) or chemical methods (through Colchicines) are employed to produce a mutant strain. Most of the time mutants are produced due to lack of particular enzyme, enzyme deficiency results in metabolic blockage at particular stage. At this stage this microorganism may accumulate with an intermediate before blockage and need artificial supply another intermediate which may arises after block. Such organisms are useful to study some biogenetic pathways. A mutant of *Lactobacillus* is source of Mevalonic acid, an important intermediate in isoprenoid compound pathway. In case of higher plants, the production of mutant strain is not successful to study the biogenetic pathways.

Applications of Tracer Techniques

Tracer techniques are importantly used to investigate the biogenetic pathways in plants to synthesize secondary metabolite. These secondary metabolites have medicinal importance in the treatment of various diseases. By knowing the biogenetic pathways one can utilize this knowledge to synthesize the important secondary metabolite by chemically or by plant tissue culture techniques. Some of the important achievements of tracer techniques are enumerated below.

- To study squalene cyclization by using radiolabeled carbon and hydrogen (^{14}C, ^{3}H) in labeled mevalonic acid.
- To study the interrelationship between 4 methyl sterols and 4,4 dimethyl sterols by using radiolabeled carbon acetate.
- Use of $2\text{-}^{14}C$ labeled mevalonate to study the biosynthesis of terpenoids via chloroplast isolated in organic solvents.
- Investigation of cinnamic acid in coumarin pathway by using radiolabeled coumarin.
- To confirm the origin of carbon and nitrogen atoms of purine by using ^{14}C or ^{15}N precursor.
- Use of ^{14}C labeled carbon dioxide to determine the sequence of formation of compounds in carbon fixation pathway in photosynthesis by using algae Chlorella.

Probable Questions

Long answer questions

1. Explain Shikimic acid pathway and its significance in detail.
2. Write in detail about amino acid synthesis.
3. Explain the biosynthetic pathway of terpenoids and steroids.
4. Describe in detail about precursor product sequence and competitive feeding.
5. Write a note on Acetate hypothesis.
6. List the basic metabolic pathways and explain Isoprenoid biosynthesis.
7. Write an account of biogenetic pathways of alkaloids from different amino acids.
8. Give a detailed view of biosynthesis of glycosides.
9. Explain in detail the use of tracer technique in biosynthetic pathway.
10. Explain any two detectors used in tracer technique

Short answer questions

1. Explain the biosynthesis of aromatic amino acid.
2. Explain biosynthesis of anthraquinone glycosides.
3. Explain biosynthesis of isoprenoids.
4. Explain the biosynthesis of triglycerides.
5. Write an isotopes and their detection methods (detectors).
6. Write a note on Sequential analysis.
7. Write a note on Geiger -Muller technique.
8. Write a note on Scintillators and its applications in the study of biosynthetic pathways.

Very short answer questions

1. What are stress compounds?
2. Define radiolabeled isotopes.
3. Enlist the amino acids produced through Shikimic acid pathway.
4. Enlist the methods used for introduction of labeled compounds in biosynthetic pathways
5. Explain grafting method.
6. Explain biosynthesis of phenolic compounds.
7. Explain biosynthesis of flavonoid aglycone.
8. Enlist the pharmaceutically important secondary metabolites with examples.
9. Write applications of tracer techniques.
10. Write the building blocks for synthesis of anthraquinone glycoside and aromatic amino acids.

Unit II

General Introduction, Composition, Chemistry & Chemical Classes, Biosources, Therapeutic uses and Commercial Applications of Following Secondary Metabolites

PCI Syllabus: General introduction, composition, chemistry & chemical classes, biosources, therapeutic uses and commercial applications of following secondary metabolites:

Alkaloids: Vinca, Rauwolfia, Belladonna, Opium

Phenylpropanoids and Flavonoids: Lignans, Tea, Ruta

Steroids, Cardiac Glycosides & Triterpenoids: Liquorice, Dioscorea, Digitalis

Volatile oils: Mentha, Clove, Cinnamon, Fennel, Coriander

Tannins: Catechu, Pterocarpus

Resins: Benzoin, Guggul, Ginger, Asafoetida, Myrrh, Colophony

Glycosides: Senna, Aloes, Bitter Almond

Iridoids, Other terpenoids & Naphthaquinones: Gentian, Artemisia, taxus, carotenoids

Book Chapter Content

- Drugs containing Alkaloids
  - Introduction
  - Vinca
  - Rauwolfia
  - Belladona
  - Opium

- Drugs containing Phenylpropanoids and Flavonoids
  - Introduction
  - Lignans
  - Ruta
  - Tea
- Drugs containing Steroids, Cardiac Glycosides and Triterpenoids
  - Introduction
  - Liquorice
  - Dioscorea
  - Digitalis
- Drugs containing Volatile oils
  - Introduction
  - Mentha
  - Clove
  - Cinnamon
  - Fennel
  - Coriander
- Drugs containing Tannins
  - Introduction
  - Black Catechu
  - Pale Catechu
  - Pterocarpus
- Drugs containing Resins
  - Introduction
  - Benzoin
  - Guggul
  - Ginger
  - Asafoetida
  - Myrrh
  - Colophony
- Drugs containing Glycosides
  - Introduction
  - Senna
  - Aloes
  - Bitter almond

- Drugs containing Iridoids, Terpenoids and Naphthaquinones
    - Introduction
    - Gentian
    - Artemisia
    - Taxus
    - Carotenoids

Drugs Containing Alkaloids

Alkaloids are secondary metabolites obtained from plant metabolism. More than 10,000 different alkaloids have been identified in species from over 300 plant families. Generally, alkaloids are derivatives of amino acid and basic in nature. Alkaloid contains generally heterocyclic ring in it and exhibit potent pharmacological activity even at low doses. Many alkaloids are poisonous if used in large doses. Most of the alkaloids have a very bitter taste. Alkaloids are secondary metabolite of plant metabolism. Their function in plant is still unknown but because of bitter taste these are natural compounds to deter herbivorous organisms.

Generally, alkaloids are colorless crystalline solids with sharp melting point. These are naturally occurring organic compounds containing basic nitrogen atoms. This nitrogen atom is situated in some cyclic system. Based on structure and nature of cyclic system alkaloids are divided in classes like, indoles, tropanes, quinolines, isoquinolines, pyrrolidines, pyridines, terpenoids and steroids. Alkaloids further can be classified by the name of families e.g. Papaverine from Papaveraceae family. Alkaloids shows variety of physiological actions like anti-inflammatory, analgesic, hepatoprotective, anaesthetic, parasympatholytic, antibacterial, hypnotic, antitumor and many more. Alkaloids can react with acids and then form salts like inorganic alkalis. Mostly the free bases of alkaloids are soluble in the organic non-polar solvents and the salts of most alkaloids are soluble in water.

Following are few important drugs containing alkaloids, their biological sources, chemical composition, therapeutic uses, and commercial applications.

Vinca

Synonym: Periwinkle, Catharanthus

Biological source: It consist of dried whole plant of *Catharanthus roseus Linn*

Family: Apocynaceae

Geographical source: The plant is native of Madagascar and found in South Africa, India, USA, Europe and Australia.

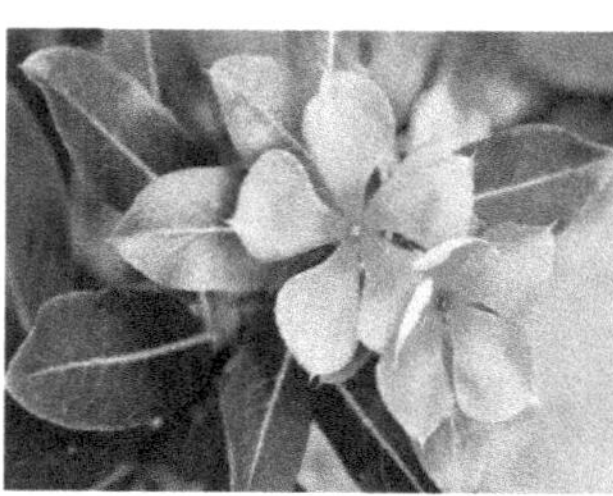

Chemical Constituents: Vinca is an Indole alkaloid containing drug. The important alkaloids are the dimer indole- indoline alkaloids vinblastine, vincristine (0.0002%), vinorelbine and vindesine which are known for their significant anticancer activity. It also consists of indole monomeric alkaloids vindoline and catharanthine. The other alkaloids present in vinca are ajmalicine, serpentine and tetrahydroalstonine. The monoterpenes, sesquiterpenes, indole and indoline glycosides are also present in vinca.

Vincristine

Vinblastine

Identification Tests

1. Vinca powder when treated with sulphuric acid and *p*-dimethyl amino benzaldehyde (Van-Urk's reagent) gives violet red color indicating the presence of Indole alkaloids.

Therapeutic uses

- Antineoplastic agent.
- Antihypertensive drug.
- Antidiabetic agent.
- The fresh flowers of the Periwinkle show gentle purgative action.
- It is used in herbal medicine as tonic in the treatment of menorrhagia and in hemorrhage.
- It is also used in the treatment of inflamed tonsils and sore throat.
- Used externally or internally for bleeding piles.

Commercial application

- Vinca is used to extract vincristine, vinblastine, vinorelbine and vindesine.
- Vinblastine as an integral part of medicinal treatment regimens for testicular carcinoma, breast cancer, germ cell tumors and both Hodgkin and non-Hodgkin lymphomas.
- Vincristine has been approved to treat acute leukemia, neuroblastoma, Wilm's tumor, Hodgkin's disease, several non-malignant hematologic disorders and other lymphomas.
- Antineoplastic activity of vindesine has been reported in acute lymphocytic leukemia, blast crisis of chronic myeloid leukemia, malignant melanoma, pediatric solid tumors and metastatic renal, breast, esophageal and colorectal carcinomas.
- It is one of the ingredients of the formulation cytocristin manufactured by Cipla.

Rauwolfia

Synonym: Sarpagandha, serpentine root, chota chand

Biological Source: Rauwolfia consists of dried roots of the plant known as *Rauwolfia serpentina* Benth.

Family: Apocynaceae

Geographical Source: Found in tropical regions of Asia, America, and Africa. Commercially cultivated in India, Myanmar, Srilanka, Thailand and America. In India it is cultivated in Bihar, Uttar Pradesh, Orissa, Tamilnadu, West Bengal, Karnataka, Maharashtra and Gujarat.

Chemical Constituents: Rauwolfia contains about 0.7–3% total alkaloidal bases from which more than 80 alkaloids have been isolated. The prominent alkaloids from rauwolfia are categorized as 1. Indole alkaloids, 2. Indoline alkaloids 3. Indolenine alkaloids 4. Oxyindole alkaloids and 5. Pseudo indoxyl alkaloids.

The important alkaloids isolated are reserpine, rescinnamine, rescidine and deserpidine. The other alkaloids are ajmaline, ajmalicine, ajmalinine, serpentine, serpentinine, tetrahydroreserpine, isoajmaline and yohimbine. Other than alkaloids, it also contains phytosterols, oleoresins, fatty acids and sugars.

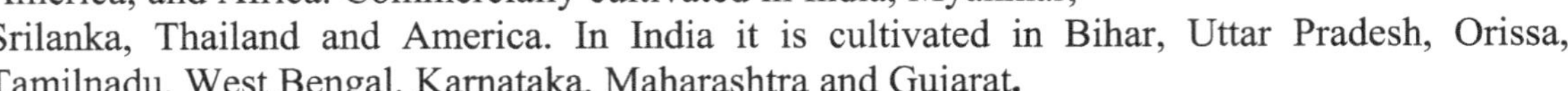

Serpentine

Reserpine

Rescinnamine

Yohimbine

Ajmalicine　　　　　　　　Ajmaline

Identification Tests

1. Rauwolfia powder when treated with sulphuric acid and *p*-dimethyl amino benzaldehyde (Van-Urk's reagent) gives violet red color indicating presence of Indol alkaloids

2. Transverse section of Rauwolfia root shows red coloration along with medullary rays when treated with concentrated nitric acid.

Therapeutic uses

- Therapeutically Rauwolfia used as Antihypertensive agent.
- Used as hypnotic sedative and tranquilizing agent.
- It is also used as an antipyretic agent.
- It can cure hysteria and insomnia.

Commercial application

- Due to its ability to lower blood pressure, commercially used in the treatment of hypertension.
- Because of tranquilizing effect, used in mild anxiety conditions and some neuropsychiatric disorders.
- Used to treat circulatory diseases, to relieve the obstruction of normal cerebral blood flow.
- Induces uterine contractions so used in difficult childbirth.

Belladona

Synonym: Belladona leaf, Deadly night shade leaf, Death's herb

Biological Source: Belladonna consists of the leaves and other aerial parts of *Atropa belladonna* Linn. known as European Belladona or *Atropa acuminata* Royle ex-Lindley known as Indian Belladona.

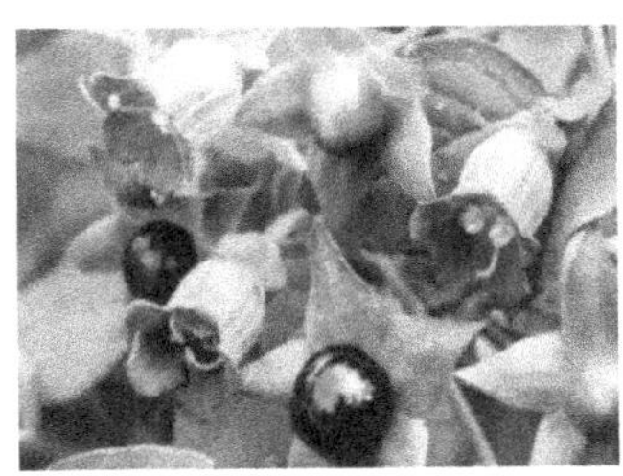

Family: Solanaceae

Geographical Source: Belladona is indigenous to England and other European countries. It is cultivated in United States, Canada, UK, Germany, and India.

Chemical Constituents: Belladona is a tropane alkaloid containing drug. It consists of 0.4 to 1 % of total alkaloid content. The percentage may vary depending on the part of the plant from 0.3 to 0.6 %. The important alkaloid present is *l*- hyoscyamine. The other chemical compounds present are atropine (racemic form of *l*-hyoscyamine), belladonine, scopoletin, hyoscine, pyridine, N- methyl pyrroline, phytosterols and volatile bases.

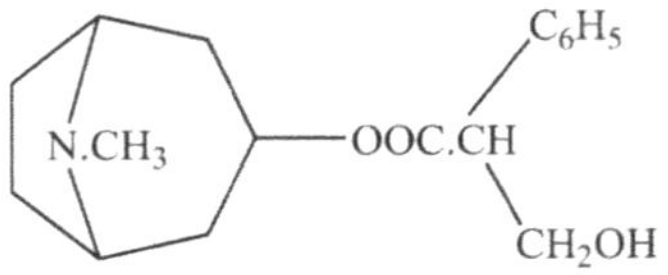

Atropine

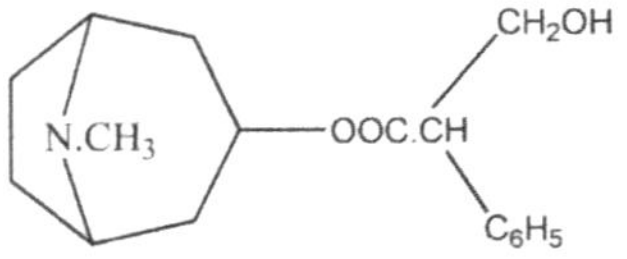

Hyoscyamine

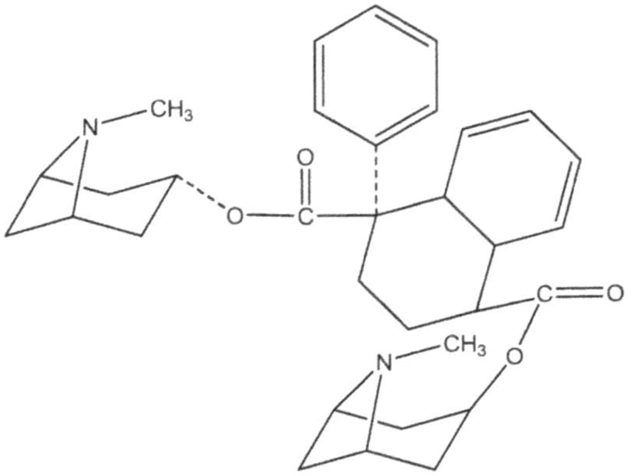

Belladonine

Identification tests

1. *Vitali Morin test*: Treat the alkaloid with concentrated nitric acid and then evaporate to dryness on water bath. To the dry nitrated residue, add 2-3 drops of acetone followed by 2-3 drops of methanolic potassium hydroxide solution. The appearance of violet color indicates the presence of tropane alkaloid.

2. To the alcoholic solution of scopoletin add ammonia solution and observe. Blue fluorescence can be observed.

Therapeutic uses

- It is parasympatholytic drug with anticholinergic activity.
- It reduces the secretions like sweat, saliva and gastric juices.
- It has purgative action.
- It has narcotic, sedative action.

Commercial application

- It is used as mydriatic and painkiller.
- Used to control excess motor activity of the GI tract and spasm of the urinary tract.

- Belladona is used as adjunctive therapy in the treatment of digestive disorders.
- It is also used as antidote in opium and chloral hydrate poisoning.

Opium

Synonym: Raw Opium, Afim

Biological source: Opium is the dried latex obtained by the incisions on unriped capsules of *Papaver somniferum* Linn.

Family: Papaveraceae

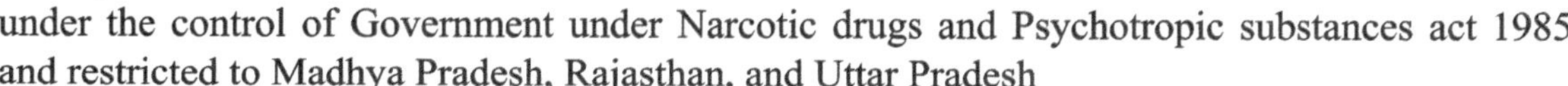

Geographical source: It is found in India, Pakistan, Afghanistan, Turkey, Russia, China, Iran and Burma. In India the cultivation is under the control of Government under Narcotic drugs and Psychotropic substances act 1985 and restricted to Madhya Pradesh, Rajasthan, and Uttar Pradesh

Chemical Constituents: Opium latex contains the alkaloids mainly derived from phenylalanine and tyrosine. Around 35 alkaloids are present, in that morphine is present around 10 to 16 %. The different types of alkaloids present in Opium are as follows.

Phenanthrene alkaloids: Morphine, codeine, pseudo morphine, thebaine, ethyl morphine. Heroin an acylated form of morphine is also present.

Benzylisoquinoline alkaloids: Papaverine, Narceine, Codamine.

Pthalide isoquinoline type alkaloids: 1-Narcotine, Noscapine.

Cryptopine type alkaloids: Protopine, cryptotropine.

It also consists of sugar, wax, mucilage, coloring matter. In Opium the alkaloids are present as salts of meconic acid.

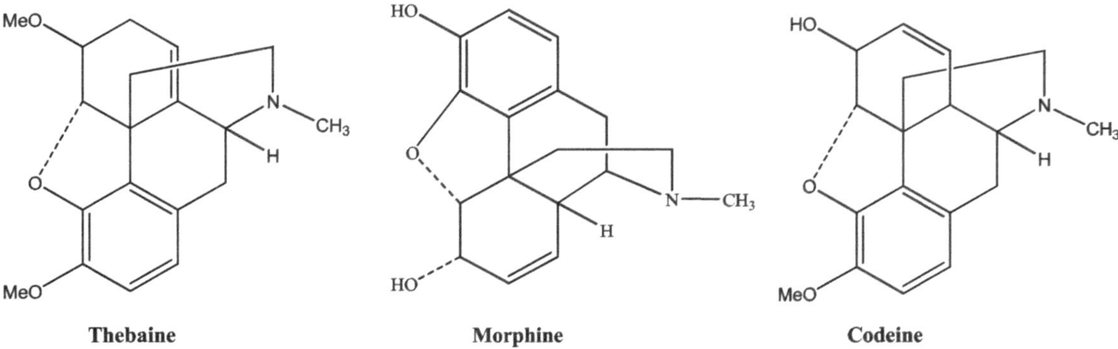

Thebaine   Morphine   Codeine

Heroin

Papaverine

Identification tests

1. To the aqueous extract of opium add ferric chloride solution. The deep reddish purple color indicates the presence of meconic acid.

2. To the morphine solution add concentrated sulphuric acid followed by formaldehyde. The dark violet color is observed.

3. Morphine when sprinkle on nitric acid produces orange red color.

Therapeutic uses

- Opium comes under the category of hypnotic, sedative, and analgesic. The activity mainly attributed to morphine.

- Codeine is antitussive agent and painkiller as well.

- Papaverine has muscle relaxant action

- Narcotine has a specific depressant action on cough reflex so act as antitussive.

Commercial applications

- Codeine is mild sedative and is used as antitussive agent in cough syrup and cough linctus.

- Morphine is used as pain killer when other pain killers are failed to reduce the pain.

- It is used in the treatment of diarrhea and dysentery.

- Papaverine is smooth muscle relaxant and is used to cure muscle spasms.

- Opium, morphine, and heroin causes addiction.

Drugs Containing Phenylpropanoids and Flavonoids

Phenylpropanoids: Phenylpropanoids are diverse group of secondary metabolites synthesized by plants from the amino acids phenylalanine and tyrosine. The structure of phenylpropanoids contains a phenyl ring attached to a three-carbon propyl side chain and devoid of nitrogen. A wide range of natural compounds comes under the phenylpropanoids. Phenylpropanoids helps the plants to adjust with the environment, protects from UV light, defend against herbivores and pathogens and mediate plant pollinator interactions. Cinnamic acid plays an important role in biosynthesis of phenylpropanoids. Phenylpropanoids are diversified as simple phenylpropanoids (e.g. Cinnamaldehyde, cinnamyl alcohol and their derivatives, cinnamic acids and their derivatives and complex phenylpropanoids), Lignoids (viz. lignans, neolignans), flavonoids and coumarins.

Flavonoids: Flavonoids are a class of phenylpropanoids synthesized in plants as a secondary metabolite. Chemically the flavonoid ring consists of 15 carbon skeleton structure containing two phenyl rings and a heterocyclic ring. Flavonoids plays important functions in plants. these are the most important plant pigments for flower coloration designed to attract pollinating agents. In higher plants flavonoids are involved in UV filtration, symbiotic nitrogen fixation or they may act as chemical messenger, physiological regulator, and cell cycle inhibitor.

Basic skeleton of Flavonoids

Lignans: Lignans are dimeric phenylpropanoid derivatives synthesized by plants as a secondary metabolite. Lignans are structurally diverse compounds and actively involved in the plant defense mechanism as antioxidants, biocides and phytoalexins. Lignans are stereospecific dimers of cinnamic alcohol bonded at carbon 8. In the plants lignans generally occur free or bound to sugars.

Lignan

Ruta

Synonym: Rue

Biological source: Ruta is the odoriferous herb *Ruta graveolens* L.

Family: Rutaceae

Geographical source: *Ruta graveolens* is native to Mediterranean region and distributed throughout the world as an ornamental herb.

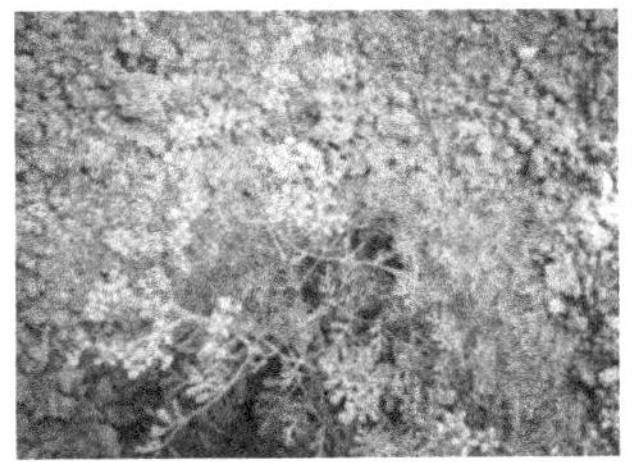

Chemical Constituents: The important active principles of the plants are flavonoid glycoside – rutin, alkaloids such as coquisagenine, gravioline, psoralens such as bergaptene and xantotoxine. It also contains essential oil. The chief constituents of essential oil are ketones, sesquiterpenoids and monoterpenoids.

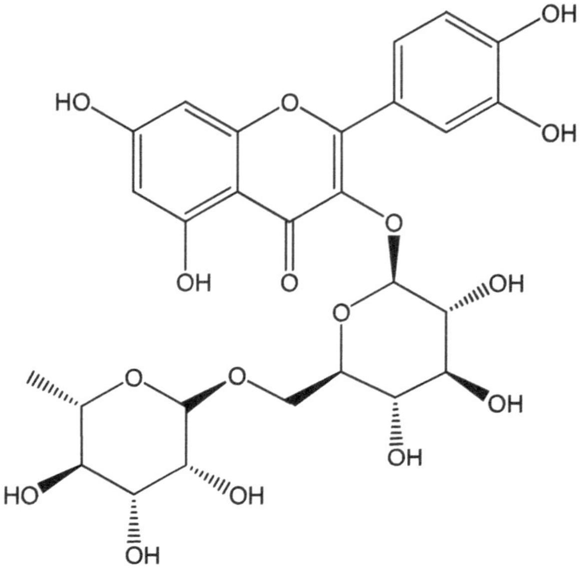

Rutin

Identification tests

1. **Ammonia test:** Filter paper dipped in the alcoholic solution of the drug powder followed by exposure to ammonia vapor. Presence of yellow spot on filter paper indicates the presence of flavonoid glycosides.

2. **Vanillin HCl test:** The alcoholic solution of the drug treated with vanillin HCl shows the presence of pink color indicating the presence of flavonoid glycoside.

Therapeutic uses

- It is used to treat strains and sprains.
- It is used to treat pain and stiffness in the hands, wrists, feet and legs.
- It is used to treat injuries of the cartilage and tendon around the joints and injuries to tissues lying over the bone.
- It is used as antispasmodic, stomachic, irritant.
- Used as an abortifacient.

Commercial application

- Rue oil is used as antirheumatic, antispasmodic agent.
- To relieve bone pains due to injuries, strains and dislocations.

- Used as emmenagogue.
- Rutin supports and strengthen the inner linings of blood vessels and reducing blood pressure.

Tea

Synonym: Camellia thea

Biological source: It consists of the prepared leaves and leaf buds of *Thea sinensis L.*

Family: Theaceae

Geographical source: Tea is cultivated in India, Srilanka, China, Indonesia and Japan.

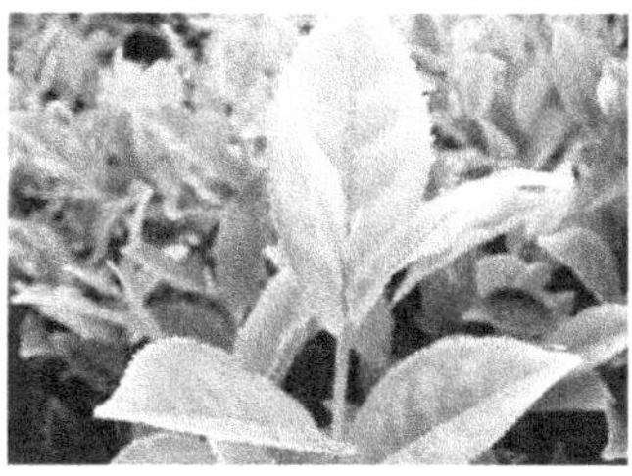

Chemical Constituents: Tea leaves are rich source of natural bioactive compounds like phenolic acids, flavonoids, coumarins, alkaloids, polyacetylenes, saponins and terpenoids. The important purine alkaloid is caffeine (1-5 %). It also contains theobromine and theophylline. The major flavanols in tea are catechin, epicatechin, epicatechin gallate, gallocatechin, epigallocatechin and epigallocatechin gallate. The color of tea leaves due to tannins and odor is due to presence of volatile oil. Tea also contains protein, wax, resin and ash in traces.

(-)-Epicatechin

(+)-Catechin

Caffeine

Identification tests

1. **Murexide test:** Purine alkaloids gives Murexide color reaction. Take caffeine crystals in petridish and add hydrochloric acid and potassium chlorate followed by heating to dryness on a water bath. Expose the residue to dilute ammonia vapors. The purple residue indicates the presence of caffeine. The purple color disappears on addition of alkali.

2. Caffeine gives white precipitate when treated with tannic acid.

Therapeutic uses

- Caffeine shows cerebral vasoconstrictor effect
- Flavanols present it tea shows strong antioxidant activity
- It acts as astringent
- It acts as diuretic

Commercial application

- Used as central nervous system stimulant due to its vasoconstrictor effect on CNS
- It has shown anticancer activity by reducing oxidative stress.
- It is also used as anti-inflammatory agent.

Drugs Containing Steroids, Cardiac Glycosides and Triterpenoids

The cardiac glycosides or steroidal glycosides are an important class of naturally occurring drugs composed of two structural features such as glycone and aglycone steroidal moieties. Chemically, the aglycone part of the cardiac glycoside is a steroidal moiety. They are either C-23 or C-24 steroids based on the presence of five membered or six membered lactone ring. If five membered lactone ring is present known as cardenolides and if six membered lactone ring is present known as bufadienolides. The lactone ring of cardenolides contains only one double bond and attached with steroidal nucleus through C-17 position. In bufadienolides the lactone ring contains 2 double bonds and is attached to steroidal nucleus through 17 β position.

Cardenolide

Bufadienolide

These cardiac glycosides increase the output force of the heart and increase the rate of contractions by acting on the cellular sodium potassium ATPase pump. These are commonly used in the treatment of congestive heart failure. The commonly used cardiac glycosides are digitoxin, digoxin and bufallin.

Steroids are degraded triterpenoids. Triterpenoids are commonly distributed in plant kingdom. They are present in either free state or esters of glycosides. They are further classified as tetracyclic triterpenoids and pentacyclic triterpenoids. These are mostly stress compounds (phytoalexins) produced by the plants due to stress.eg. Azadirachtin from *Azadirachta indica.*

Liquorice

Synonym: Yasti, mulethi, radix glycyrrhizae

Biological source: It consist of dried, unpeeled roots and stolons of *Glycyrrhiza glabra* Linn

Family: Leguminosae

Geographical source: Commercially cultivated in Spain, England, Iraq, China, India, Turkey and United States.

Chemical Constituents: The chief constituent of Liquorice is triterpenoid saponin known as glycyrrhizin (6-8%) which is potassium and calcium salt of glycyrrhizinic acid. Glycyrrhizin is 50 times sweeter than sucrose. Glycyrrhizinic acid on hydrolysis yields glycyrrhetinic acid which has triterpenoid structure. Liquorice also contains the flavonoids liquirtin and isoliquirtin. The yellow color to drug is due to isoliquirtin. The drug also contains sugar, starch (29%), protein, fat, resin aspargin, yellow coloring matter in outer part of the root, and volatile oil in traces.

Glycyrrhetinic acid

Identification tests

The deep yellow color is produced when 80% of sulphuric acid is added to a thin section or powder of Liquorice due to conversion of flavones glycoside liquirtin to isoliquirtin.

Therapeutic uses

- Reduces throat irritation and has expectorant and demulcent action.
- Due to mineralocorticoid activity it is used in the treatment of chronic inflammation like rheumatoid arthritis and addison's disease.
- It is used as an antispasmodic.
- It has antigastric effect so used in the treatment of peptic ulcers.
- It is also used as an antibacterial agent.

Commercial application

- Liquorice is used as a flavouring agent in formulations

- It is used as a sweetening agent in pharmaceutical preparations.

- Liquorice due to saponin content also used as foam stabilizing agent.

- Liquorice is used in the formulations to potentiate the effect of senna.

- Externally the roots are used in the treatment of herpes, eczema and skin infections.

Dioscorea

Synonym: Yam

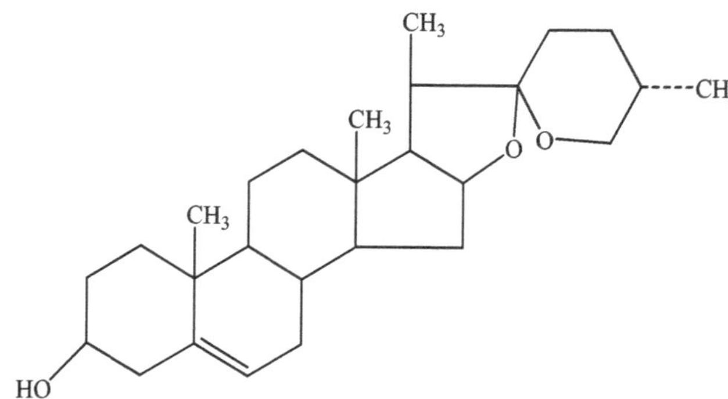

Biological source: It consists of dried tubers of the plants, *Dioscorea deltoida, D.floribunda, D. compositae* and other several species of Dioscorea.

Family: Dioscoreaceae

Geographical source: Dioscorea mainly found in North America, Mexico, China and India. In India it is mainly found in Kashmir, Punjab and Himachal Pradesh upto an altitude of 1000 to 3000m.

Chemical Constituents: The dioscorea rhizomes contain dioscin which have diosgenin as aglycone part (4 to 6 %) and is a steroidal sapogenin. Other glycosides present are hecogenin, smilagenin, epismilagenin and beta isomer yammogenin. It also contains 75% starch and an enzyme sapogenase. The steroids present in dioscorea are cholesterol, stigmasterol and P- sitosterol.

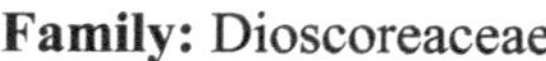

Diosgenin

Identification tests

1. **Libermann Burchard's Test**: To the drug solution in acetic anhydride, add few drops of concentrated sulphuric acid. The color changes to reddish violet followed by green color.
2. **Salkowski Test**: To the chloroform extract of the drug add few drops of concentrated sulphuric acid. Chloroform layer produces red color indicating the presence of steroids.

Therapeutic uses

- Dioscorea showed effect of reducing the serum cholesterol level.

- Diosgenin in wild yam has also been known to have beneficial effects at controlling blood pressure and cholesterol levels.

Commercial application

- Rhizomes are rich source of diosgenin – a steroidal moiety.

- Diosgenin is most widely used as an active ingredient in preparation of many steroid drugs, sex hormones and oral contraceptive pills.

- Diosgenin is used for the commercial synthesis of cortisone, pregnenolone, progesterone, and other steroid products.

- Cortisone prepared from diosgenin is used in the treatment of rheumatic diseases and ophthalmic disorders

Digitalis

Synonym: Foxglove leaves

Biological source: Digitalis consists of dried leaves of *Digitalis purpurea* Linn.

Family: Scrophulariaceae

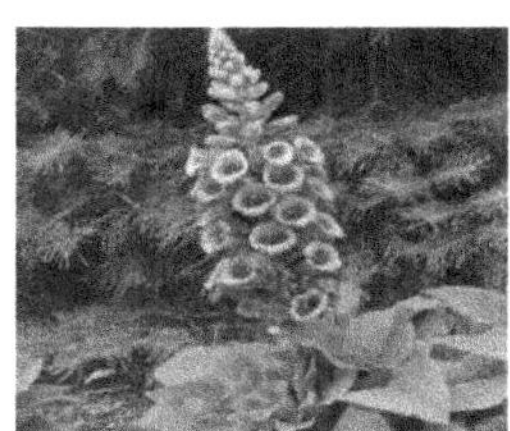

Geographical source: It is cultivated in England, Germany, France and other parts of Europe, United States, India.

Chemical Constituents: Digitalis leaves consists of 0.2 to 0.45 % mixture of both primary and secondary glycosides. The primary metabolites are less absorbed and less stable compared to secondary glycosides, Purpurea glycosides A and B and glucogitoloxin are primary glycosides. Purpurea glycosides A and B are present in fresh leaves and can undergo enzymatic hydrolysis to give digitoxin and glucose or gitoxin and glucose respectively. Digitalis also contains many other glycosides like, odoroside H, gitaloxin, verodoxin and glucoverodoxin. The saponins present in leaves are digitonin, tigonin and gitonin. The flavone present is luteolin which is responsible for the color of the leaves.

Identification tests

1. **Keller- Kiliani Test:** 1gm of the powdered leaves are extracted with 10 ml of 70% alcohol for 2 to 3 min. The extract is filtered and to 5 ml of filtrate 10 ml of water and 0.5 ml of strong solution of lead acetate is added. The filtrate is shaken with 5 ml of chloroform. Chloroform layer is separated in a porcelain dish and evaporated to yield the extract. The extract is dissolved in glacial acetic acid and a drop of ferric chloride solution is added followed by the addition of sulphuric acid. A reddish-brown color is seen in between two liquids and the upper layer becomes bluish green.

2. **Baljet Test:** To a thick section of digitalis leaf sodium picrate reagent is added. Appearance of yellow to orange color indicates the presence of glycosides.

3. **Legal Test:** The extract is dissolved in pyridine and sodium nitroprusside solution is added and made alkaline. Appearance of pink or red color indicates the presence of glycoside.

Purpurea Glycoside A $\xrightarrow{\text{Enzymatic hydrolysis}}$ Digitoxin + Glucose

↓ hydrolysis

Gitoxigenin + 3- Digitoxose

Purpurea Glycoside B $\xrightarrow{\text{Enzymatic hydrolysis}}$ Gitoxin + Glucose

↓ hydrolysis

Gitoxigenin + 3- Digitoxose

Digitoxigenin

Digitoxin

Therapeutic uses

- Digitalis has a cardiotonic activity and commonly used in the treatment of congestive heart failure.

- Digitalis is used as diuretic in cardiac edema.

- Digitalis can increase blood flow throughout the body and reduce swelling in hands and ankles.

Commercial application

- Commercially digitalis leaves are used to isolate digoxin.

- Commercially used in the treatment of congestive heart failure, atrial fibrillation, atrial flutter in the form of tablets or capsules

Drugs Containing Volatile Oils

The odorous and volatile principles of plant and animal sources are known as volatile oils. They are liquid in nature and will evaporate or volatilizes when exposed at an ordinary temperature hence called as ethereal oil. They represent the essence or concentrated constituents of the crude drug so also known as essential oil. Volatile oils are generally secreted in oil cells, in secretion ducts in glandular hairs or in cavities. These are generally mixtures of hydrocarbons and oxygenated compounds derived from these hydrocarbons. Many types of organic compounds found in volatile oil viz. hydrocarbons, alcohol, ketones, aldehydes, ethers, oxides, esters and others. The odor and taste of the volatile oil is mainly due to oxygenated compounds. Volatile oils are soluble in alcohol, ether and other lipid solvents and practically insoluble in water. Volatile oils are characterized by high refractive indices and optical activity. Some important drugs from this category are discussed below.

Mentha

Synonym: Mint, peppermint oil

Biological source: Mentha consists of Aerial parts of plant *Mentha piperita* Linn, *M spicata* and volatile oil known as peppermint oil is obtained by the steam distillation of fresh aerial parts of the plants.

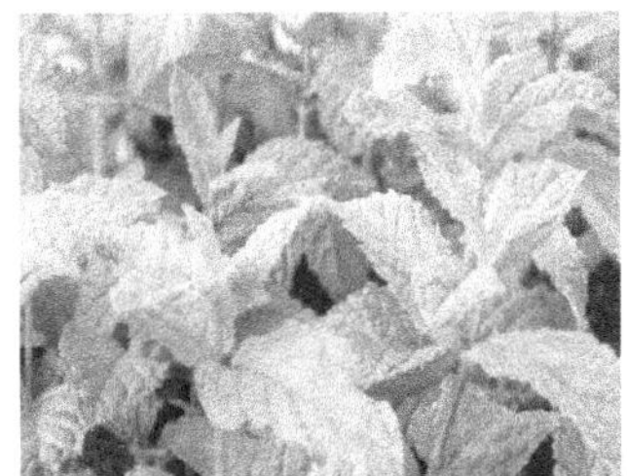

Family: Labiateae or Lamiaceae

Geographical source: It is cultivated in Europe, Japan, England, France, USA and Bulgaria. In India it is cultivated near Jammu and Uttar Pradesh.

Chemical Constituents: Mentha leaves typically consists of 1.2 to 3.9 % of essential oil with more than 300 identified components. It comprises of 52% of monoterpenes and 9 % of sesquiterpenes. Other than this it also consists of aldehydes, aromatic hydrocarbons, lactones and alcohols. In monoterpenes Menthol is the major constituent (around 70 %). It also contains menthone, methyl acetate, eucalyptol, isomenthone, menthofuran, neomenthol and limonene. In sesquiterpene β- caryophyllene is the major constituent. Many other terpene derivatives like l-limonene, isopulgeone, cineole, pinene, camphene also present. The esters such as menthyl acetate are responsible for typical minty flavor.

Carvone	Cineole	Limonene	β-Caryophyllene

Pulegone	Menthol	Menthone

Identification tests

1. Mix few drops of peppermint oil with 5 ml of nitric acid solution (prepared by 1 ml of nitric acid to 300 ml of glacial acetic acid) followed by heating on water bath. The appearance of blue color within five minutes which on further heating shows copper colored fluorescence further turns to golden yellow indicates the presence of menthol.

Therapeutic uses

- It is traditionally used as a carminative, stimulant and aromatic.
- It has counter irritant activity.
- It is a strong antioxidant agent.
- It has insecticidal activity.
- Peppermint oil shows cytotoxic effect and hence used as anticancer agent.
- It has antimicrobial activity.

Commercial application

- Commercially used as flavoring and antiseptic agent in oral hygiene products like toothpaste, tooth powders, mouth washes and gargles.
- Also used in manufacturing of chewing gums, candies, jellies, perfumes and essences.

Clove

Synonym: Clove bud, caryophyllum

Biological source: It consists of the dried flower buds of *Eugenia caryophyllus* Thumb.

Family: Myrtaceae

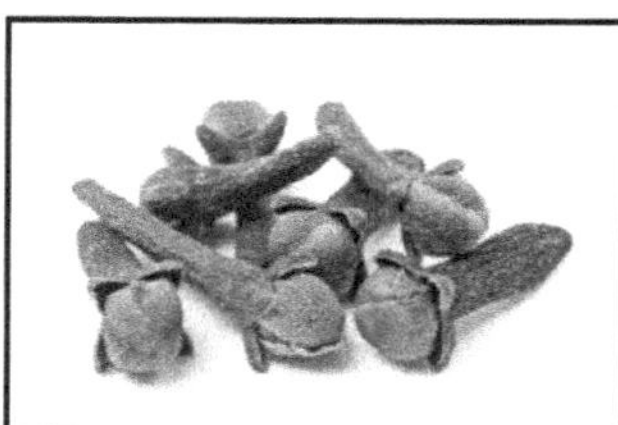

Geographical source: Clove tree is native of Indonesia. It is now cultivated chiefly in Zanzibar, Pemba, Penag, Brazil, Madagascar, Srilanka and India. In India it is mainly cultivated in Tamilnadu and kerala.

Chemical Constituents: The clove bud consists of 14 to 18 % of volatile oil. The chief constituent of volatile oil is Eugenol (around 72 to 90 %). The other components of volatile oil are acetyl eugenol, β- caryophyllene and vanillin. Clove also consists of tannins such as bicomin, methyl salicylate, gallotonic acid, kaempferol, gums, resins, fibers and several sesquiterpenes.

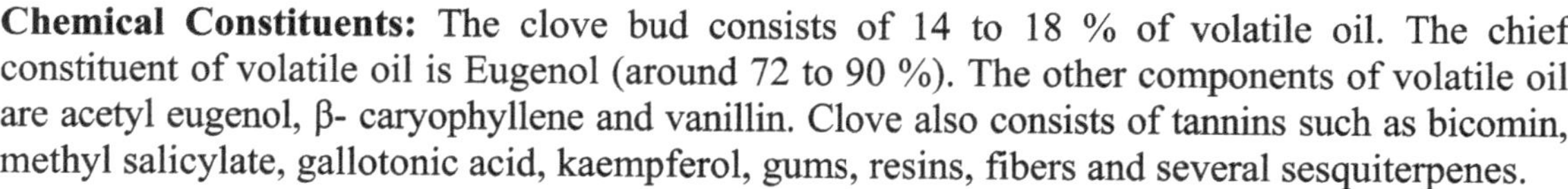

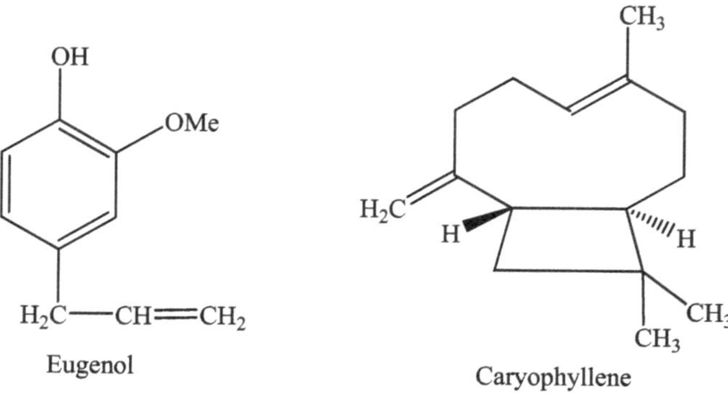

Eugenol

Caryophyllene

Identification tests

1. The transverse section of volatile oil is treated with strong potassium hydroxide solution shows the occurrence of needle shaped potassium eugenate crystals.
2. Dissolve 0.2ml of clove oil in alcohol and add ferric chloride solution. The occurrence of blue color indicates the presence of phenolic group.

Therapeutic uses

- Clove is used as dental analgesic.
- It is commonly used as carminative, stimulant and aromatic.
- It shows antimicrobial activity.
- Used in the treatment of sore throat and cough.

Commercial application

- The oil is used in perfumery and in manufacturing of vanillin.
- As a condiment in spices.
- Clove oil is used in cosmetics and pharmaceutical industry.

Cinnamon

Synonym: Kalmi dalchini, cinnamon bark

Biological source: It consists of dried inner bark of shoots of coppiced trees of *Cinnamomum zeylanicum* Nees.

Family: Lauraceae

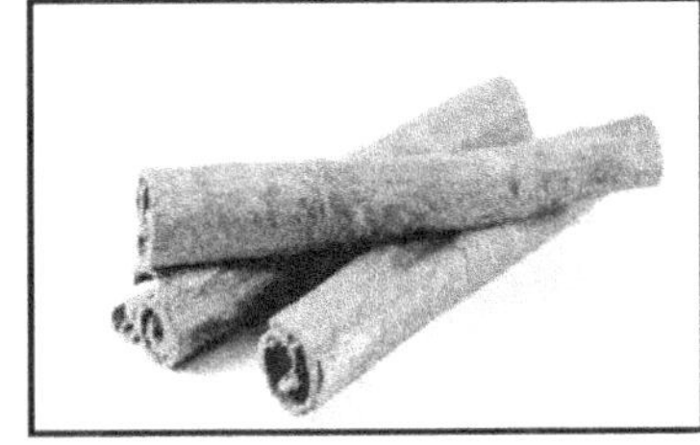

Geographical source: Cinnamon is native of Sri Lanka and found in Java, Sumatra, West Indies, Brazil, Jamaica, Mauritius and India.

Chemical Constituents: Cinnamon bark contains 0.5 to 1.2 % of volatile oil. Volatile oil contains 50 to 60 % of Cinnamaldehyde along with 5-10% of eugenol, terpene hydrocarbons and small quantities of ketones and alcohols. Bark also contains tannins (phlobatannins), mucilage, calcium oxalate, and mannitol (sugar).

Cinnamaldehyde

Cinnamic acid

Eugenol

Identification tests

1. Dissolve a drop of cinnamon oil in 5 ml of alcohol and add a drop of ferric chloride solution. Appearance of pale green color indicates the presence of cinnamaldehyde and eugenol. Eugenol gives blue color with ferric chloride while cinnamaldehyde gives brown color resulting in formation of pale green color after few minutes.

2. Treat the alcoholic extract of cinnamon bark with phenylhydrazine hydrochloride; appearance of red color indicates the presence of cinnamaldehyde.

Therapeutic uses

- Cinnamon bark is used as carminative, stomachic and mild astringent.
- Used as an analgesic, antirheumatic, antispasmodic.
- It has antifungal and antibacterial activity.

Commercial application

- Commercially it is used as a flavoring agent in pharmaceuticals.
- It is used as condiment and spice.
- Also used in perfume industry.
- It is used in the dentifrices and candy preparations.
- Used in manufacturing of candy and bakery products.

Fennel

Synonym: Sounf, Fennel fruits, Fructus foeniculli.

Biological source: It consists of dried ripe fruits of *Foeniculum vulgare* Miller.

Family: Umbelliferae

Geographical source: Fennel plants are indigenous to Mediterranean countries of Asia and largely cultivated in Germany, France, Japan, Russia, Romania and India.

Chemical Constituents: The fennel fruit consists of 4 to 5 % of volatile oil and the chief constituents of volatile oil are anethole - a phenolic ether (50-60 %) and a ketone- fenchone around 20 %. The oil also shows the presence of β-pinene, anisic acid, phellandrine and anisaldehyde. Fruits also consists of 20 % of fats and proteins.

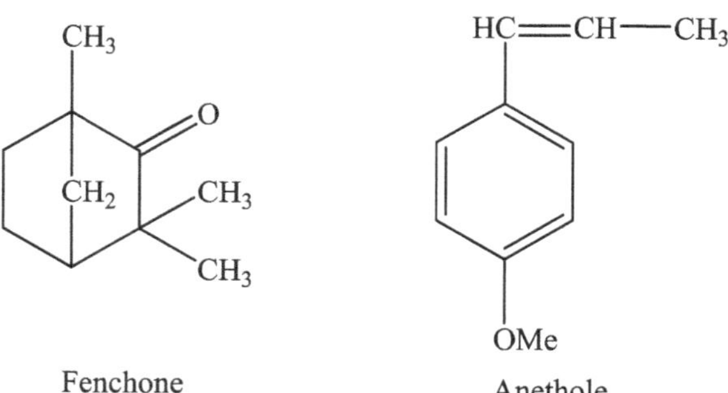

Fenchone

Anethole

Identification tests

1. To the thin section of fennel add a drop of Sudan Red III, appearance of red color shows the presence of volatile oil.
2. Alcoholic extract of fennel when treated with vanillin sulphuric acid reagent; color changes to yellow orange indicating the presence of volatile oil.

Therapeutic uses

- Fennel is used as stomachic, diuretic and as a digestive.
- Fruits are used as carminative, aromatic and stimulant.
- It is also used as antispasmodic, antipyretic and antimicrobial agent.
- It has expectorant activity as well as anti-inflammatory activity.

Commercial application

- Volatile oil of fennel is the major ingredient of many gripe waters used as an antispasmodic in infants
- Fennel oil is used as flavoring agent in pharmaceutical and food industry.

Coriander

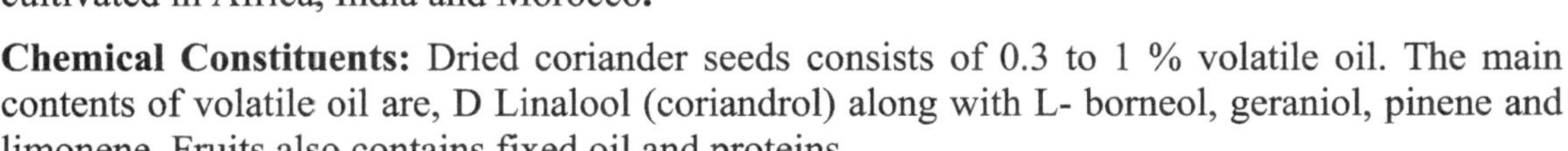

Synonym: Coriander fruits, cilantro

Biological source: It consists of dried riped fruits of *Coriandrum sativum* Linn.

Family: Umbelliferae

Geographical source: Coriander is cultivated throughout European countries mainly in Russia and Hungary ad Holland. It is also cultivated in Africa, India and Morocco.

Chemical Constituents: Dried coriander seeds consists of 0.3 to 1 % volatile oil. The main contents of volatile oil are, D Linalool (coriandrol) along with L- borneol, geraniol, pinene and limonene. Fruits also contains fixed oil and proteins.

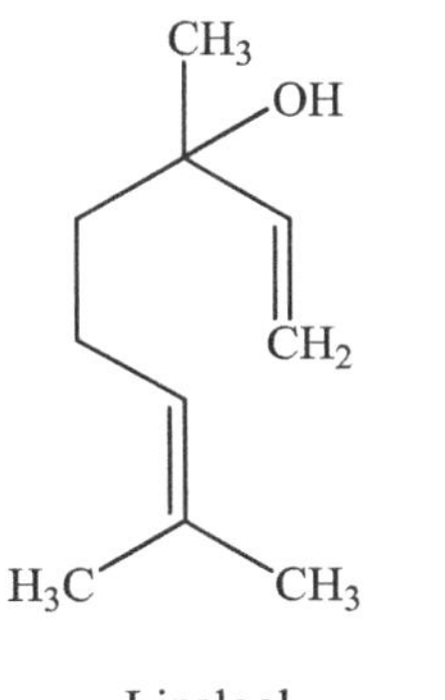

Linalool

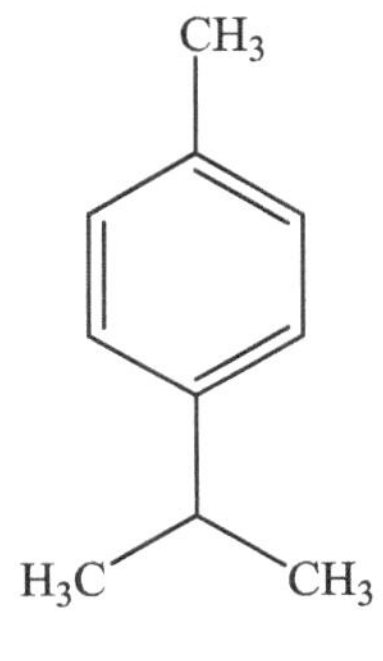

p-Cymene

Identification tests

1. To the thin section of coriander add a drop of Sudan Red III, appearance of red color shows the presence of volatile oil.

2. Alcoholic extract of coriander when treated with vanillin sulphuric acid reagent; color changes to yellow orange indicating the presence of volatile oil.

Therapeutic uses

- The coriander fruits as well as volatile oil is used as carminative, aromatic and stimulant.

- Coriander oil is used to prevent gripping along with purgatives.

- Fruits are used as diuretic, appetizer and stomachic.

Commercial application

- It is ingredient of compound spirit of orange and cascara elixir.

- It is used as condiment and spice.

Drugs Containing Tannins

Tannin term is derived from the French "tannin" which means tanning agents. Tannins are complex organic non nitrogenous plant products which generally have astringent properties, widely distributed in the plant kingdom. Previously the term was applied to chemicals which were used to combine with proteins of animals hide to convert them into leather which is known as tanning of the hide. Hence tannins are substances which are detected by tanning test due to its absorption on standard hide powder. The test is known as Goldbeater's skin test.

Some of the low molecular weight tannins do not respond to Goldbeater's skin test are known as pseudo tannins. Broadly tannins can be defined as the derivatives of polyhydroxy benzoic acid capable of combining with proteins. Tannins are alcohol and water-soluble compounds. They cause precipitation of proteins and alkaloids. Tannins react with ferric salts and imparts dark blue or green color with ferric salt. Important examples from this category are discussed here.

Catechu

Black Catechu

Synonym: Cutch, Kattha, Khadir

Biological source: Black catechu is the dried aqueous extract prepared from the heartwood of *Acacia catechu* Wild.

Family: Leguminosae

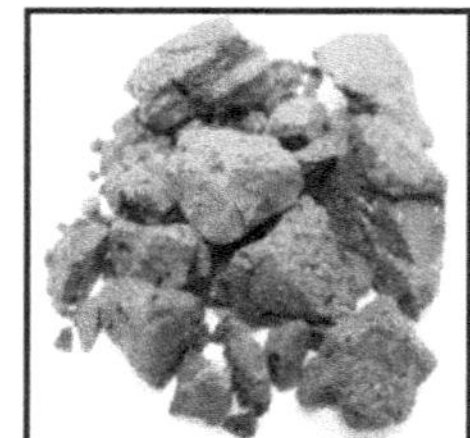

Geographical source: Black Catechu is a traditional plant of India and found in Punjab, Assam, Madhya Pradesh, Maharashtra, Gujarat, Rajasthan, Bihar and Tamilnadu.

Chemical constituents: Black catechu contains 2 to 10% of Acacatechin which undergoes oxidation in presence of water to form catechutanic acid which constitutes about 25 to 33 % of the drug. It also contains gum, catechin red, quercetin and its derivatives.

(+)-Catechin

Identification tests

1. Powder of black catechu when treated with vanillin and hydrochloric acid; shows pink or red color due to presence of catechin.

2. *Match stick test*: Dip the match stick in hydrochloric acid then in extract of black catechu and heat near the flame. Matchstick burns with purple or magenta color as catechin reacts with hydrochloric acid to produce phloroglucinol which burns along with lignin to give purple color.

3. Aqueous extract of black catechu if treated with lime water produces brown color which on standing forms red precipitate.

4. Treat the black catechu aqueous solution with ferric chloride solution gives bluish black color indicating the presence of tannins.

Therapeutic uses

- Black catechu is used as an astringent for cooling and digestive purpose.
- It is used to treat the itching of throat, mouth gums.
- Used to treat cough.
- It causes contraction of guts so used to treat diarrhea.

Commercial application

- Black catechu is used in the manufacturing of herbal tooth powders.
- It is used in formulation of lozenges.
- Used in dyeing and tanning industry.

Pale Catechu (Gambier)

Synonym: Gambier, catechu

Biological Source: Pale catechu consists of a dried aqueous extract prepared from the leaves and young twigs of *Uncaria gambier* Roxburgh.

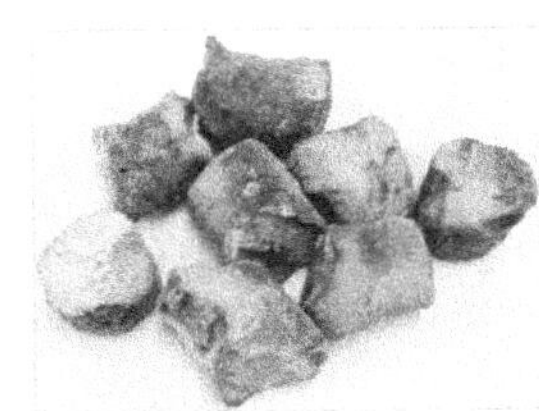

Family: Rubiaceae

Geographical source: Pale catechu is cultivated in Malaysia, Singapore, Sumatra and Indonesia.

Chemical Constituents: Pale catechu contains 7-33 % of catechin, 22% of catechutanic acid, flavonoids like quercetin, catechu red. Gambierfluorescin is a fluorescent substance. It also shows presence of pyrogallol, fixed oil and waxes.

(+)-Catechin

Identification tests

1. Powder of pale catechu when treated with vanillin and hydrochloric acid; shows pink or red color due to presence of catechin.

2. *Gambier fluorescin test*: Extract powder drug with alcohol. To the alcoholic extract add sodium hydroxide and shake with petroleum ether, shake well and allow it to stand for few minutes. Petroleum ether layer emits green fluorescence indicating the presence of gambierfluorescin. Black catechu gives this test negative.

3. *Matchstick test*: Dip the matchstick in hydrochloric acid followed by in extract of black catechu and heat near the flame. Matchstick burns with purple or magenta color as catechin reacts with hydrochloric acid to produce phloroglucinol which burns along with lignin to give purple color.

4. Chloroform extract of the drug in white porcelain dish shows green yellow color due to presence of chlorophyll. Black catechu gives this negative.

Therapeutic uses

* Pale catechu is used as an astringent for cooling and digestive purpose.
* Used to treat cough.
* It causes contraction of guts so used to treat diarrhea.

Commercial application

* Commercially used in dyeing and tanning industry.

Pterocarpus

Synonym: Malabar Kino, Indian Kino tree, Rakta chandan

Biological source: It consists of dried juice obtained by making vertical incisions to the stem bark of the plant *Pterocarpus marsupium* Linn.

Family: Leguminosae

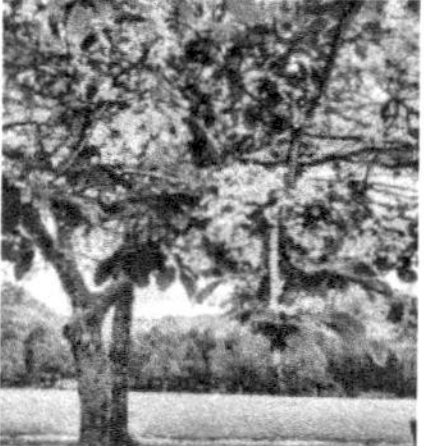

Geographical source: Pterocarpus is a traditional drug found in hilly regions of India viz. Gujarat, Uttar Pradesh, Bihar, Orissa and in forests of Assam, Kerala, West Bengal.

Chemical Constituents: Pterocarpus contains kinotannic acid (70 to 80 %), kino red and catechol, resin and gallic acid. Kinnotanic acid is non glucosidal tannin and kino red is anhydride of kinoin. Kinoin is insoluble phlobaphene and is derived by the action of oxydase enzyme.

Kinotanic acid

Identification tests

1. To the aqueous solution of pterocarpus add ferrous sulphate solution, appearance of green color indicates the presence of tannins.
2. To the aqueous solution of pterocarpus add any alkali like potassium hydroxide; violet color appears.
3. Treat the pterocarpus extract with mineral acid, precipitate is formed.

Therapeutic uses

- Pterocarpus is used as an astringent.
- Used in the treatment of diarrhoea and dysentery, toothache.
- Used as antidiabetic in ayurveda.

Commercial application

- It is commercially used in the manufacturing of Ayurvedic dental preparations.
- Used as antidiabetic in traditional system of medicine.

Drugs Containing Resins

Resins are the complex amorphous product of more or less solid characteristics containing mixtures of essential oil, oxygenated products of terpenes and carboxylic acids which on heating first sets softened and then melt. These are found as an exudate from the trunk of various trees. Resins are produced and stored in schizogenous or schizolysigenous glands of the plants. The resin and its products are marketed as unorganized drugs. These are insoluble in highly polar (water) and highly nonpolar (petroleum ether) solvents but soluble in alcohol, solvent ether, benzene or chloroform. Resins are naturally occurring but are now commonly prepared synthetically.

Benzoin

Siam Benzoin

Synonym: Gum Benzoin

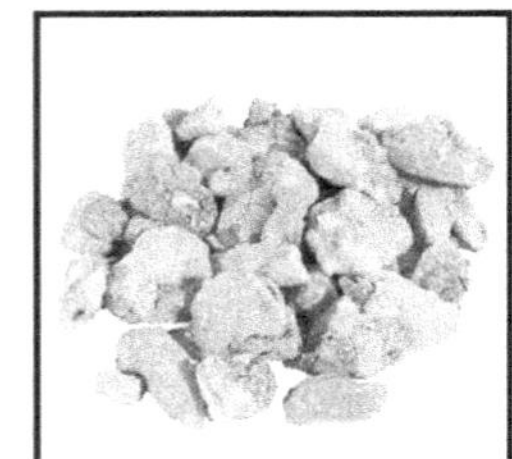

Biological Source: Siam benzoin is a balsamic resin obtained from stems of *Styrax tonkinensis* Craib.

Family: Styracaceae

Geographical Source: Siam benzoin cultivated in Thailand, North Vietnam, Annam and North Laos.

Chemical Constituents

The important chemical constituent of Siam Benzoin is Coniferyl benzoate approximately 60 to 80 %. The other constituents are free benzoic acid, vanillin, benzyl cinnamate and triterpene derivatives like siaresinolic acid.

Coniferyl benzoate

Identification tests

1. Add 2 to 3 drops of sulphuric acid to the petroleum ether solution of Benzoin in a evaporating dish. Siam benzoin shows purple red color while Sumatra Benzoin produces reddish brown color.
2. Take Alcoholic solution of Benzoin and add few drops of ferric chloride solution. A green color appears in case of Siam Benzoin due to the presence of phenolic compound coniferyl benzoate. In case of Sumatra Benzoin this test is negative.

Therapeutic uses

- Siam Benzoin is used as antiseptic, expectorant.
- It is used as antioxidant in cosmetics.
- It acts externally as a protective agent.

Commercial application

Siam benzoin commercially used in the cosmetic preparation as an antioxidant and protective.

Sumatra Benzoin

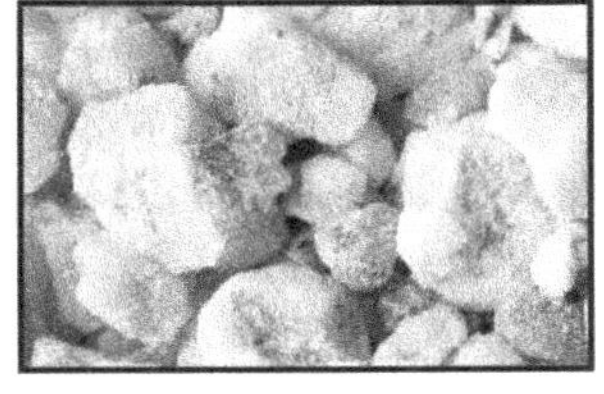

Synonym: Loban, Benzonium

Biological source: Sumatra Benzoin is obtained by the incisions on the stems of *Styrax benzoin* Drynder, and *Styrax parallel-neurus* Perkins.

Family: Styracaceae

Geographical source: The trees are cultivated in Sumatra, Java, Malaya and Borneo.

Chemical Constituents: The chief chemical constituent of Sumatra Benzoin is free balsamic acids mainly cinnamic and benzoic acids and their esters. The drug also shows the presence of triterpenic acids like siaresinolic acid, sumaresinolic acid, traces of vanillin, phenyl propyl cinnamate, cinnamyl cinnamate and phenylethylene.

Siaresinolic acid

Identification tests

1. Add 10 % of aqueous solution of potassium permanganate to the benzoin powder. Sweet smell is produced due to oxidation of Cinnamic acid present in Sumatra Benzoin. This test comes negative for Siam Benzoin.

2. Add 2 to 3 drops of sulphuric acid to the petroleum ether solution of Benzoin in a evaporating dish. Siam benzoin shows purple red color while Sumatra Benzoin produces reddish brown color.

3. Take Alcoholic solution of Benzoin and add few drops of ferric chloride solution. A green color appears in case of Siam Benzoin due to the presence of phenolic compound coniferyl benzoate. In case of Sumatra Benzoin this test is negative.

Therapeutic uses

- Sumatra Benzoin is used as antiseptic and expectorant.
- It is used as an antioxidant.

Commercial application

- It is used in perfume industry
- It is used in cosmetic preparations.

Guggul

Synonym: Gum Guggul, scented bdellium

Biological source: Guggul is oleogum resin obtained by incision method on the bark of *Commiphora mukul* Hook and *Commiphora weightii* Bhand.

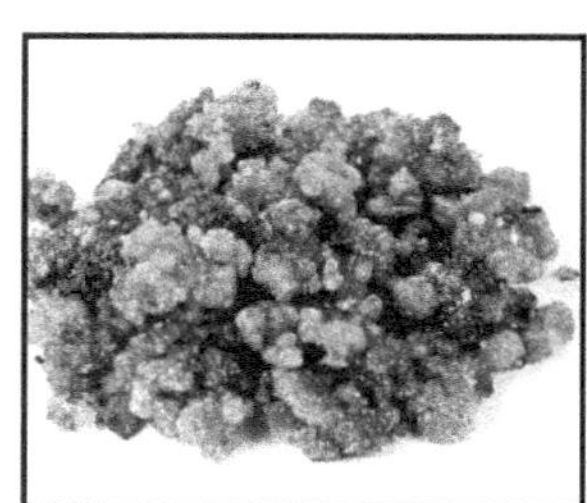

Family: Burseraceae.

Geographical source: Guggul is found in dry areas of India, Pakistan, Baluchistan and Arabia. In India it is cultivated in Rajasthan, Gujarat, Karnataka and Maharashtra.

Chemical Constituents: Guggul consists of approximately 60% of gum, 30 % resin 1 to 1.5 % volatile oil and 5 to 6 % moisture. The gum contains sterols mainly guggulsterols I to VI, sitosterol, cholesterol, E and Z guggulsterone, sugars and amino acids.

E-guggulsterone

Z-guggulsterone

Identification tests

1. Extract the guggul resin with ethyl acetate, to the extract add acetic anhydride followed by boiling on water bath. Cool the solution and add few drops of sulphuric acid. Green color develops at the junction indicating the presence of steroids.

Therapeutic uses

- Guggul has anti-inflammatory activity.
- It has hypolipidemic and hypocholesteremic activity hence used in the treatment of obesity.
- It has strong antirheumatic activity.
- Used as antiseptic, expectorant.

Commercial application

- It is the traditional medicine and used in the manufacturing of Ayurvedic guggul formulations like kanchnar guggul, guggul yog.
- Used in the treatment of obesity.

Ginger

Synonym: Zingiber, Saunth

Biological source: Ginger consists of fresh or dry rhizomes of *Zingiber officinale* Roscoe.

Family: Zingiberaceae

Geographical source: Ginger is found in South East Asia and cultivated mainly in India, west indies, Africa, Australia Taiwan and Mauritius.

Chemical constituents: Ginger contains about 1 to 2 % of volatile oil, pungent resinous matter around 5 to 8 % and starch in abundant amount. Volatile oil consists of zingiberene, gingerol, shogals, sesquiterpene derivatives. The pungency and aroma of ginger is attributed to gingerol which is yellow in color.

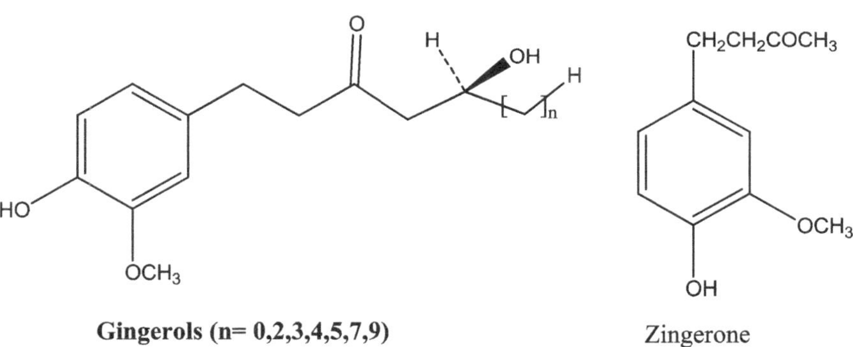

Gingerols (n= 0,2,3,4,5,7,9)   Zingerone

Identification tests

1. Boil the aqueous extract of ginger with 2 % potassium hydroxide solution. The ginger loses its pungency.

Therapeutic uses

- Ginger is used as stomachic, digestive and carminative.
- It is used as stimulant and antipyretic.
- It is used as aromatic and flavoring agent.
- It is used in the treatment of dyspepsia, vomiting, spasms.
- Used as a household remedy to treat cough, cold, sore throat and headache.
- It has antihistaminic activity hence used to treat allergic conditions.

Commercial application

- Used in many traditional ayurvedic formulations like Sitopaladi churna, Trikau churna.
- Used as flavoring agent in pharmaceuticals.
- Used in the formulations of lozenges, candies and toothpaste.

Asafoetida

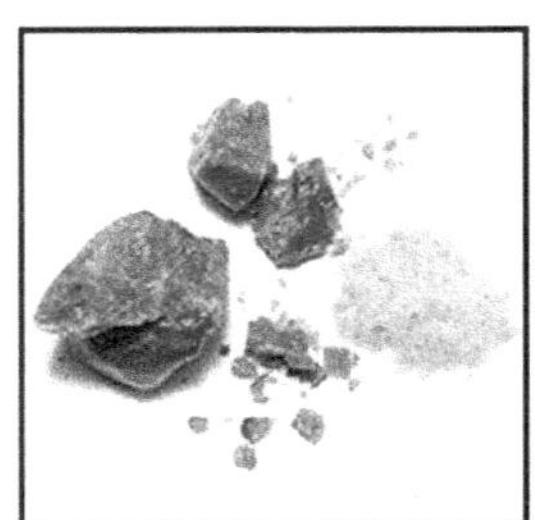

Synonym: Hing, Devil's dung

Biological source: Asafoetida is an oleogum resin obtained as an exudate by giving incisions on decapitated roots and rhizomes of *Ferula foetida* Royel, *Ferula rubricaulis* Boiss and other species of Ferula

Family: Umbelliferae

Geographical source: It is found in Afghanistan, Persia and Iran.

Chemical constituents: Asafoetida consists of 40 to 60 % of resin, 20 to 25 % gum and 4 to 20 % volatile oil. The resin of the drug contains asaresinotanol in combination with ferulic acid. The odour of the asafoetida is due to presence of sulphur compounds. It also contains complex mixture of sesquiterpene umbelliferyl ethers generally with monocyclic or bicyclic terpenoids moiety. Resin consists of ester of asaresinotannol and ferulic acid. Ferulic acid on treatment with hydrochloric acid get converted into umbelliferone.

Umbellic acid

Umbelliferone

Identification tests

1. Asafoetida if triturated with water forms milky emulsion.
2. Boil 0.5 gm of asafoetida with hydrochloric acid for few minutes. Filter and add ammonia to the filtrate. A blue fluorescence is observed due to conversion of ferulic acid to umbeliferone.
3. Add few drops of 50% nitric acid on fractured surface of drug, green color can be observed.
4. Add few drops of sulphuric acid on fractured surface of the drug, a red color can be observed which changes to violet on washing with water.

Therapeutic uses

- Asafoetida is used as carminative, anti-spasmodic and intestinal antiseptic.
- Used as an enema for intestinal flatulence.
- Used in chronic asthma, bronchitis and whooping cough.

Commercial application

- Used as a condiment in spices.
- Used as flavouring agent.
- Used in veterinary medicines.

Myrrh

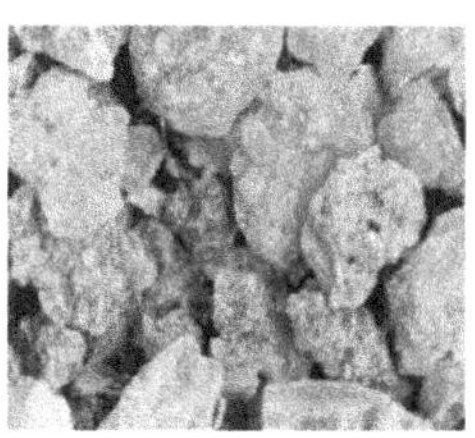

Synonym: Bol, Gum Myrrh

Biological source: Myrrh is an oleogum resin obtained from the stem of *Commiphora molmol* Eng. and other species of Commiphora.

Family: Burseraceae

Geographical source: It is found in North East Africa and Southern Arabica.

Chemical Constituents: Myrrh contains gum (55 to 61 %), resin (25 to 40 %) and volatile oil about 10 %. Resin contains ether soluble resin acids α, β and γ-commiphoric acids. It also contains volatile oil; the chief content of volatile oil are terpenes, cuminic aldehyde, eugenol, cresol, pinene, diterpene and sesquiterpenes. It also shows the presence of phenolic compounds pyrocatechin and protocatechuic acid. The unpleasant odour of the gum is due to disulphide. The gum contains proteins, carbohydrates and enzyme oxidase.

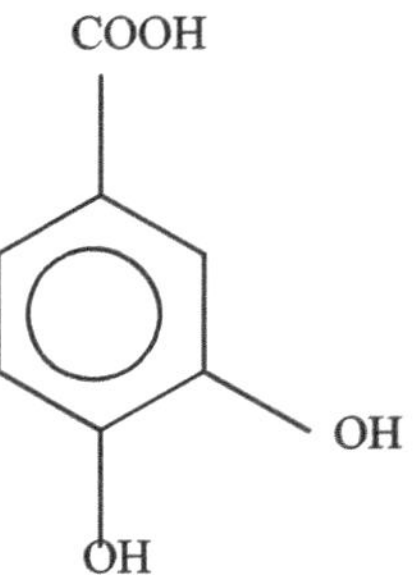

Protocatechuic acid

Identification tests

1. Triturate the powdered myrrh with water; a yellow brownish emulsion can be observed.

2. Triturate myrrh with ether, filter and evaporate. A thin film can be observed which turns red with bromine vapours and becomes purple with nitric acid.

Therapeutic uses

- It acts an antiseptic and stimulant.
- It has astringent property.
- It is antiinflammatory and protective in nature.
- It is used in treatment of asthma and bronchitis.

Commercial application

- Commercially used in the formulation of tooth powder, mouth washes and gargles due to its astringent property
- Alcoholic extract is used as fixative in perfumery industry.

Colophony

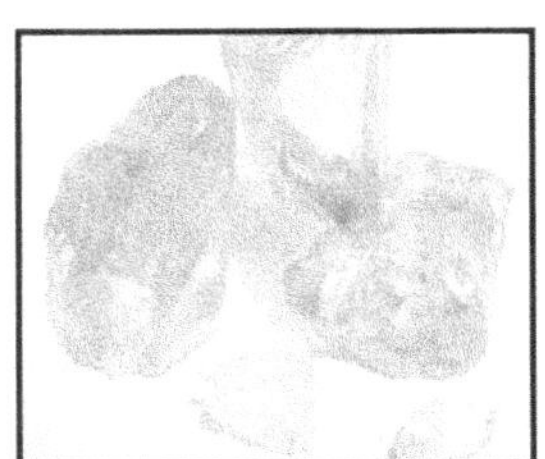

Synonym: Amber resin, Pine resin

Biological source: Colophony is a solid residual mass left after distillation of the volatile oil from the oleoresin from the plant *Pinus palustris* and other species of *Pinus*.

Family: Pinaceae

Geographical source: The *pinus* tress are widely cultivated in united states, France, Italy, Spain, China, Pakistan and India. Colophony is mainly produced in United States and contributes around 80% of world supply.

Chemical Constituents: Colophony contains about 90% resin acids known as abietic acid, resins and fatty acid esters. It shows the presence of mixture of dihydroabietic acid and dehydroabeitic acid, It also contains sipinic acid and a hydrocarbon.

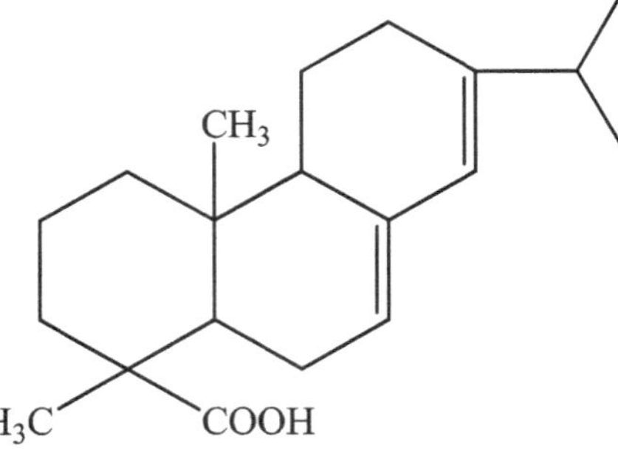

Abietic acid

Identification tests

1. Dissolve powdered colophony in acetic anhydride and add one drop of sulphuric acid. Shake it well. The purple color appears which rapidly changes to violet.

2. The alcoholic solution of colophony turns blue litmus to red due to acid.

3. Dissolve colophony in petroleum ether (60-80) and filter. Shake the filtrate with twice the volume of it with 0.15% (W/V) cupric acetate solution. The organic layer shows emerald green color due to formation of copper salt of abietic acid.

Therapeutic uses

* Colophony is stimulant and diuretic.

* Abietic acid shows antimicrobial, antiulcer and cardiovascular activity.

Commercial application

* Colophony used in the pharmaceuticals for the preparation of zinc oxide plasters, ointments and other adhesive plasters.

* It is commonly used in the manufacture of printing inks, rubber, dark varnishes, sealing wax and thermoplastic floor tiles.

Drugs Containing Glycosides

Glycosides are the organic compounds of plant and animal origin which on either acidic or enzymatic hydrolysis yields one or more sugar moieties and a non-sugar moiety. Sugar moiety is known as **glycone** while non sugar moiety is known as **aglycone**. Glycone and aglycone moieties are joined by a linkage known as **glycosidic linkage** or **glycosidic bond**. The glycone and aglycone portions can be chemically separated by hydrolysis in the presence of acid. There are also numerous enzymes that can form and break glycosidic bonds. Glycosides are crystalline or amorphous substances and are soluble in water or alcohols and insoluble in organic solvents like benzene and ether. The aglycone part is soluble in organic solvents like benzene or ether. They are optically active. Glycosides do not themselves reduce Fehling's solution, the simple sugars which they produce on hydrolysis will do so with precipitation of red cuprous oxide. The sugars present in glycoside are of two isomeric forms, that is, α form and β form, but all the natural glycosides contain β-type of sugar. The therapeutic activity of glycoside is attributed to the aglycone part. The glycone part acts as a carrier.

The few representative examples of drugs containing glycosides are discussed here.

Senna

Synonym: Alexandrian Senna, Tinnevelly Senna, Senna Folia.

Biological source: Senna consists of dried leaflets of *Cassia angustifolia* Vahl. Known as Tinnevelly senna or Indian senna and *Cassia acutifolia* Delile. known as Alexandrian senna.

Family: Leguminosae

Geographical source: Indian senna is indigenous to southern Arabia and cultivated mainly in Tinnevelly and Ramnathpuram district of Tamilnadu. It also found in Sindh and Punjab region. Alexndrian senna is indigenous to South Africa. It is cultivated in Egypt, upper region of Nile river and also in Sudan.

Chemical Constituents: Senna consists of anthraquinone types of glycosides; sennoside A and sennoside B which is responsible for its purgative activity. Sennoside A and sennoside B are stereoisomers of each other. It also shows the presence of sennoside C and D. It also contains rhein, emodin, aloe emodine, rhein-8-glucoside, aloe emodin-8-glucoside, anthrone diglucoside, kaempferol and isorhamnetin. It also contains phytosterols, mucilage, resin, myricyl alcohol, salicylic acid, chrysophanic acid and calcium oxalate.

Physcion

Chrysophanol

Rhein

Aloe emodin

Sennoside A

Sennoside B

Identification tests

1. **Borntrager test for anthraquinone glycosides:** Boil the leaves with dilute sulphuric acid and filter it. To the filtrate add organic solvent like benzene, ether or chloroform and shake well and keep aside for few minutes, the organic layer is separated. To this add ammonia solution, the ammonical layer takes pink color indicating the presence of anthraquinone glycosides.

Therapeutic uses

- Senna leaves are used as laxative. The anthraquinone glycosides of senna first get absorbed in intestinal tract after which the aglycone part is separated and excreted in colon. These excreted anthraquinone irritate and stimulate the colon thereby movements are increased due to colon action. The increase in peristalsis also causes reduction in the water absorption which results in soft and bulky feaces.

- Senna is stimulant cathartic and exerts its action by increasing the tone of the smooth muscles in large intestine.

Commercial application

- Senna is commercially used as laxative in many proprietary medicines like Softovac, Laxatin

Aloes

Synonym: Kumari, Aloes

Biological source: Aloe consists of dried juice of the leaves of any of the following

Aloe barbadensis Mil. / *Aloe vera* Lin.- Curacao aloes

Aloe perryi Baker- Socotrine aloes

Aloe ferox Miller/ *Aloe Africana* Miller/ *Aloe spicata* Baker – Cape aloes.

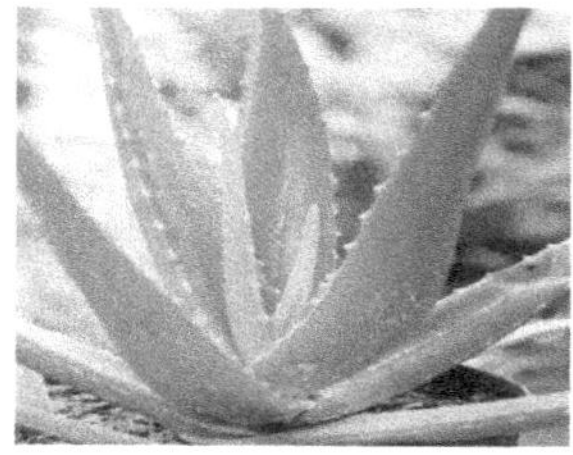

Aloe juvenna- Zanzibar aloes.

Family: Liliaceae

Geographical source: Most of the species of aloe are indigenous to South Africa. In Africa it grows in Cape colony and on the islands of Socotra and Zanzibar. In India it is cultivated throughout but commercially in North West Himalayas.

Chemical Constituents: All varieties of aloes contain three isomers of Aloins; barbaloin, β-barbaloin and isobarbaloin which constitutes crystalline aloin present around 10-30 %. Barbaloin also present in all varieties which is bitter, slightly yellow colored water soluble glycoside. Isobarbaloin is present in Curacao aloe and in traces in cape aloe while absent in Socotrine and Zanzibar aloe. Socotrine and Zanzibar aloe contains Barbaloin and β- barbaloin as chief constituent. The other constituents of aloes are rhein, emodin, aloe emodin and chrysophenol.

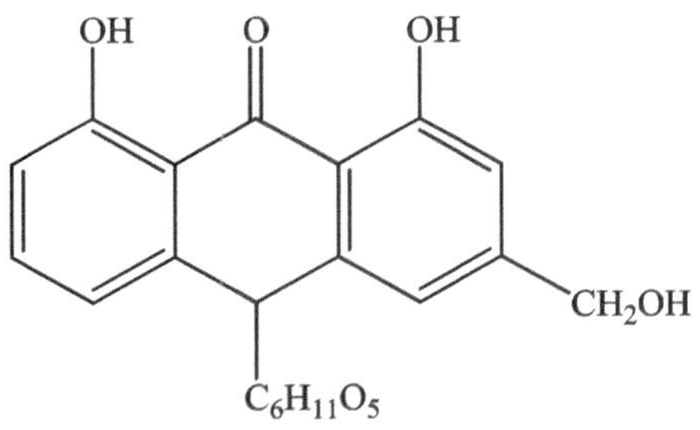

Barbaloin

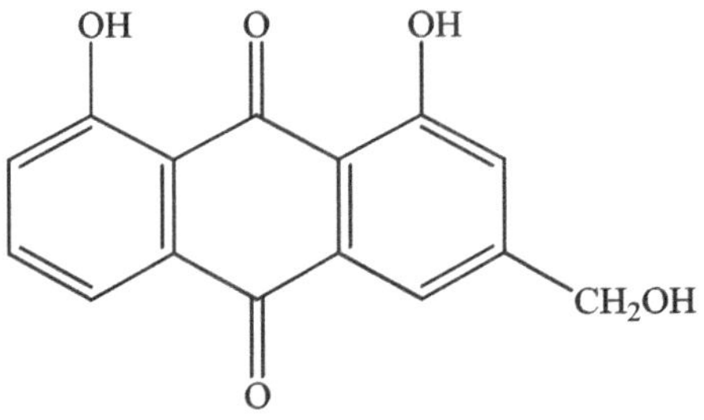

Aloe-emodin

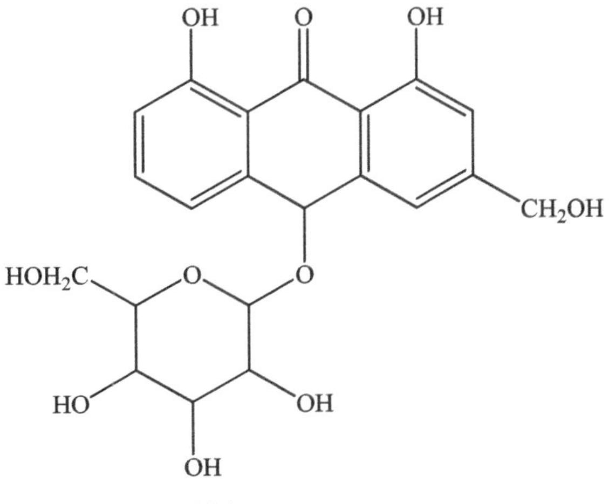

Aloin

Identification tests: Prepare 1% aqueous solution of aloes. To it add 1 gm of Kieselguhr, stir it well and filter the solution. Use this filtrate as a test solution for the identifications tests;

Table 2.1 Chemical tests for various Aloes

S.No.	Test	Cape aloe	Curacao aloe	Socotrine aloe	Zanzibar aloe
1.	Heat 2 ml of the test solution with 0.2gm of borax add this solution to a test tube containing water. A green fluorescence is produced indicating the presence of aloe emodin	Positive	Positive	Positive	Positive
2.	Take 2 ml of test solution and to it add equal quantity of freshly prepared bromine water. A pale-yellow precipitate if tetrabromalion is observed	Positive	Positive	Positive	Positive
3.	Take 5 ml of test solution and to this add 2ml of nitric acid.	Brown to green color	Reddish orange color	Pale brownish color	Yellowish brown color
4.	Cupraloin Test: 1 ml of the aloe solution is diluted to 5 ml with water and to it add 1 drop of copper sulphate solution. Bright yellow color is produced which on addition of 10 drops of saturated solution of sodium chloride changes to purple and the color persist if 15–20 drops of 90% alcohol is added.	A faint color	Wine red color	Negative	Negative
5.	Modified Borntrager's test: Take 0.1 gm of drug and add 5 ml of ferric chloride solution and 2 ml of dilute hydrochloric acid. Heat this solution on boiling water bath for 5 minutes. Cool and shake with any organic solvent like benzene. Separate benzene layer and to separated benzene layer add equal volume of dilute ammonia. A pink red color is produced in benzene layer	Positive	Positive	Positive	Positive

Therapeutic uses

- Aloe is used as irritant purgative internally.
- It acts as emollient, emmenogogue, stimulant, stomachic and tonic.
- It acts as antibacterial and soothing agent.
- It is used to treat the skin burns, skin disorders and wounds.
- It acts as antiageing agent due to its strong antioxidant activity.
- In higher doses acts as abortifacient.
- Aloe vera juice is used to treat menstrual disorders.

Commercial application

- Commercially aloe vera juice is used as antiageing agent in cosmetics

- It is used as protective and emollient in many cosmetic formulations

- It is used in skin creams to reduce inflammation, burn spots

- Pure aloe vera juice is used to maintain menstrual health of women

Bitter Almond

Synonym: Amygdala amara

Biological source: Bitter almond consists of dried ripe seed of *Prunus amygdalus* Batsch.

Family: Rosaceae

Geographical source: Bitter almond is indigenous to Iraq and Asia Minor. these are cultivated in many countries like France, Italy, Portugal, South France, Morocco and Sicily.

Chemical constituents: Bitter almond contains about 40 to 50 % of fixed oil, 20 % of proteins, mucilage and an enzyme emulsion. It also contains colorless crystalline cyanogenetic glycoside amygdalin (1 to 3 %). Amygdalin undergoes hydrolysis in presence of water and enzyme emulsion and decomposes to benzaldehyde and hydrocyanic acid. The fixed oil of bitter almond is bland in taste with slight odor. It contains olein with traces of glycerides of oleic, linoleic, palmitic, myristic and other acids.

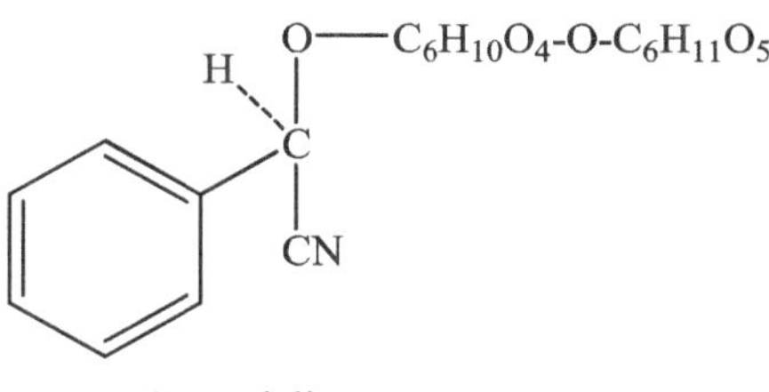

Amygdalin

Identification tests

1. *Ferriferocyanide test*: Take 1 gm of powdered drug and macerate with 5 ml of alcoholic potassium hydroxide (5 %w/v) for 5 to 7 minutes. Transfer it to an aqueous solution containing ferrous sulphate (2.5 % w/v) and heat at 60 to 70 °C for 10 minutes. Then transfer to 20 % hydrochloric acid. The appearance of distinct prussian blue color confirms the presence hydrocyanic acid.

Therapeutic uses

- Bitter almonds are used as sedative due to hydrocyanic acid content.

- The oil is used as a demulcent in skin lotion.

- It is also used in the preparation of amygdalin and bitter almond water.

Commercial application

- Commercially bitter almonds oil is used in perfumery industries.

- Fixed oil is used in skin cosmetic preparations.

Drugs Containing Iridoids, other Terpenoids and naphthaquinones

Irridoids are derivatives of monoterpenes and generally occurs as glycosides. The name derives from Iridomyrmex- a genus of ants which produces these compounds as a defensive secretion. Structurally they are cyclopentanopyran monoterpenoids. These are secondary metabolites and are plant protectants, useful as a marker for many plant species. Irridoids provides biogenetical link between terpenes and alkaloids. After the cleavage of cyclopentane ring of the iridoids secoirridoids are formed. The irridoids produced by plants primarily acts as a defense against herbivores or against infection by microorganisms. Irridoids has a wide range of bioactivities like, cardiovascular, anti-inflammatory, antispasmodic, antitumor, antiviral and immunomodulatory activities.

Naphthaquinones are products of bacterial and fungal as well as high-plants secondary metabolism. Juglone, lawsone, and plumbagin are the most widespread compounds. Naphthoquinones display very significant pharmacological properties like they are cytotoxic, antibacterial, antifungal, antiviral, insecticidal, anti-inflammatory, and antipyretic. Naphthoquinones are structurally related to naphthalene and are characterized by their two carbonyl groups in the 1,4 position, and as such, are named 1,4-naphthoquinones. Carbonyl groups may also be present at the 1,2 position, with minor incidence. Naphthoquinones are highly reactive organic compounds, used as natural or synthetic dyes whose colors range from yellow to red. These compounds and their derivatives are α,β-unsaturated carbonyl compounds. The conjugation between carbonyl and double bonds give rise to 1,4-naphthoquinone, which has an intense coloration.

The representative drugs from this category are described below.

Gentian

Synonym: Gentiana, Radix Gentianae, Kutaki

Biological source: Gentian consists of dried partially fermented roots and rhizomes of *Gentiana lutea*

Family: Gentianaceae

Geographical source: Gentian is perennial herbaceous tree indigenous to central and southern Europe.

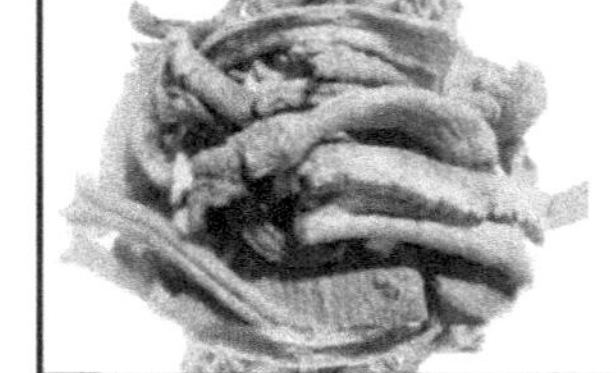

Chemical Constituents

The drug consists of bitter glycosides mainly gentiopicrin commonly known as gentiopicroside. The other glycosides are gentiamarin, gentian, amarogentin, amaroswerin, gentioside and mixture of gentiopicrin and gentisin known as gentinin. The bitter taste of the gentian is because of amarogentin. In the natural resources amarogentin is considered as bittermost substance as it imparts bitter taste even after 5.8 lakh times dilution. These glycosides contain monoterpene iridoids. The drug contains flavonoid alkaloids gentianine. It also contains free sugars, gentianose, sucrose, enzymes, yellow coloring matter, pectin, and an oil.

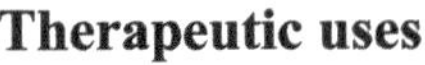

Gentiopicrin

Gentisin

Identification tests

1. The gentian extract under UV radiation shows light blue fluorescence.

Therapeutic uses

- It is generally used as bitter tonic in anorexia and dyspepsia.

- It is used as appetite stimulant.

Commercial application

- Commercially gentian is used as appetizer.

Artemisia

Synonym: Worm weed, Sweet Annie

Biological source: It consists of herb *Artemisia annua* Linn

Family: Asteraceae

Geographical source: It is a Chinese traditional herb and also found in Europe and America. It is cultivated in Vietnam, Iran, turkey and Australia.

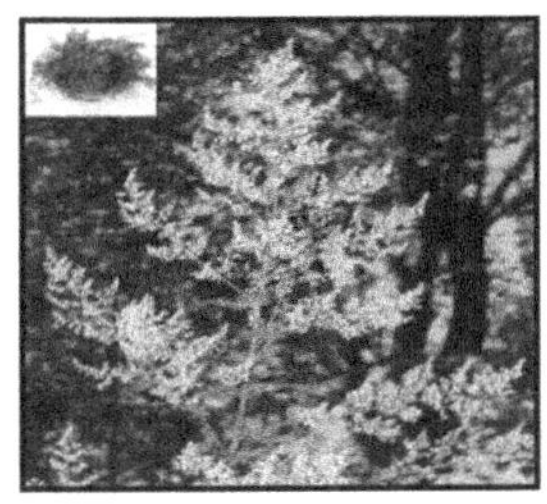

Chemical Constituents: Artemisia contains a sesquiterpene lactone artemisinin and deoxyartemisinin. It also contains, Artemisinic acid, arteanuin A and B, amyrin, luteolinstigmasterols and β- sitosterols. Volatile oil with Artemisia alcohol, Artemisia ketone, camphor, caryophyllene and myrcene also found in the drug.

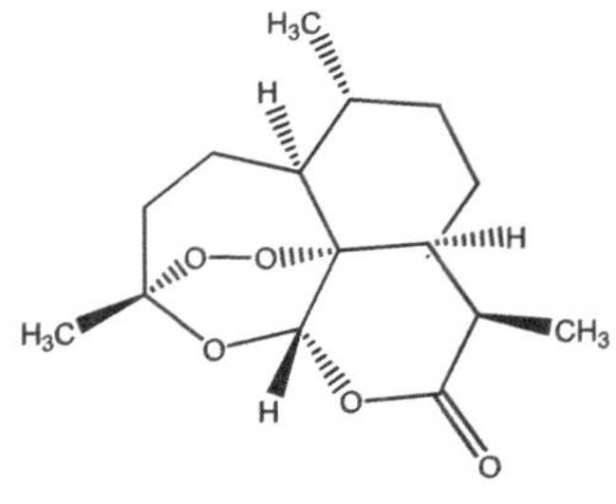

Artemisinin

Therapeutic uses

- Artemisinin is antimalarial drug against plasmodium species.

- It acts against both chloroquine sensitive and resistant *P. falciparum* and *P. vivax* malarial parasites.

- It also shows anti -HIV activity.

Commercial application

- Commercially Artemisia plant is used for the isolation of artemisinin on large scale for the treatment of malaria.

Taxus

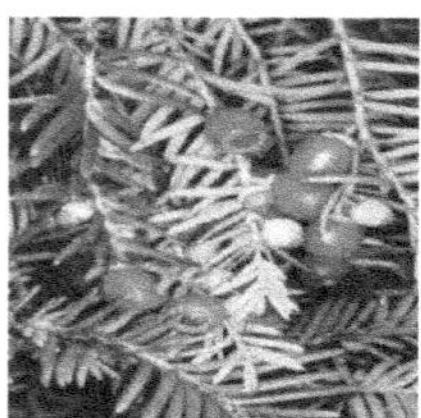

Synonym: Talispatra, Himalayan yew.

Biological source: Taxus consists of dried leaves, bark and roots of various species of *Taxus Viz.*

Taxus baccata leaves (European yew)

Taxus brevifolia stem bark (Pacific yew)

Taxus cuspidate leaves (Japanese yew)

Taxus wallichiana.

Family: Taxaceae

Geographical source: It is found in India, America and Canada.

Chemical Constituents: The chief constituent of Taxus is taxol (Paclitaxel) specially found in leaves, roots and bark. It shows the presence of baccatin, 10-deacetyl baccatin III, cephalo mannine, and baccatin III.Taxane alkaloids, diterpenoids with taxane skeleton, lignans, biflavonoids, steroids, sugar derivatives and diterpenes possessing tropone skeleton are commonly found.

Taxol

Therapeutic uses

- It has cytotoxic action so used as an anticancer agent.
- It is used as analgesic, antipyretic, antiinflammatory and anticonvulsant.

Commercial application

- Taxol is USFDA approved drug for the treatment of refractory ovarian cancer, small cell lung carcinoma, gastric and cervical cancer and carcinomas of head, neck, prostate and colon.

Carotenoids

Carotenoids are the tetraterpenoids which are yellow, orange and red organic pigments. These are produced by plants, algae, bacteria and fungi. These are lipid soluble pigments. Carotenoids can be produced from fats and other basic organic metabolic building blocks by all organisms. Around 1100 carotenoids are identified and categorized as follows.

1. Xanthophylls

2. Carotenes

Both the types of carotenoids act as an antioxidant and some can be converted into Vitamin A. Pro vitamin A carotenoids are alpha carotene, Beta carotene and beta cryptoxanthin. Non provitamin A carotenoids are lutein, zeaxanthin and lycopene.

Xanthophylls: Xanthophylls generally contains yellow pigments. They protect us from the sunlight and mostly related to eye health. Lutein and zeaxanthin comes under the category of xanthophylls. Examples of xanthophylls containing foods are spinach, pumpkin, Kale and corn.

Carotenes: These are purely hydrocarbon and contain no oxygen and associated with orange pigments. They help in growth of the plants. Beta carotene and lycopene falls under the category of carotenes. Examples of carotene containing foods are tomatoes, carrots, papaya and sweet potatoes.

All are the derivatives of the tetraterpenes and are formed from 8 isoprene molecules and contains 40 carbon atoms. Generally, tetraterpenes absorb wavelengths ranging from 400 to 550 nm (violet to green light) which causes compounds to be deeply colored yellow, orange and red.

α–carotene

β– carotene

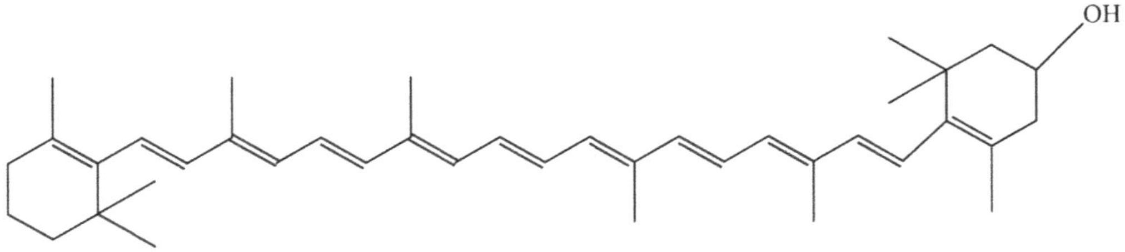

β– cryptoxanthin

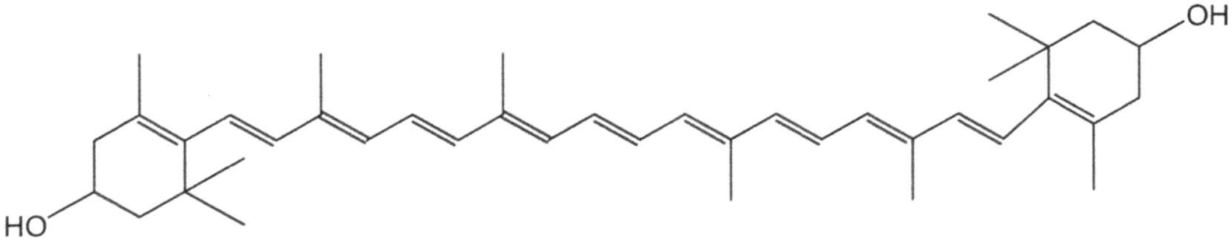

lutein

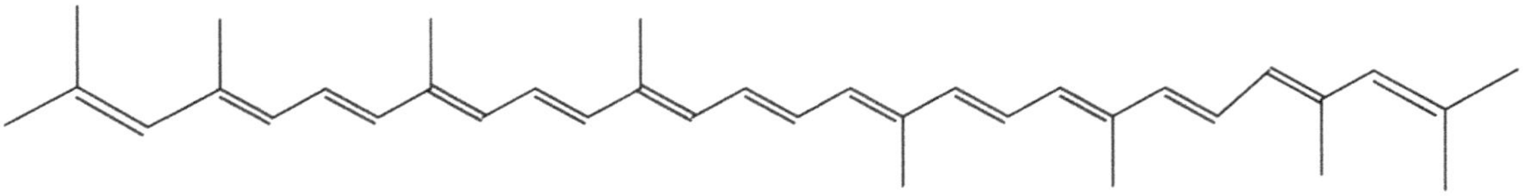

lycopene

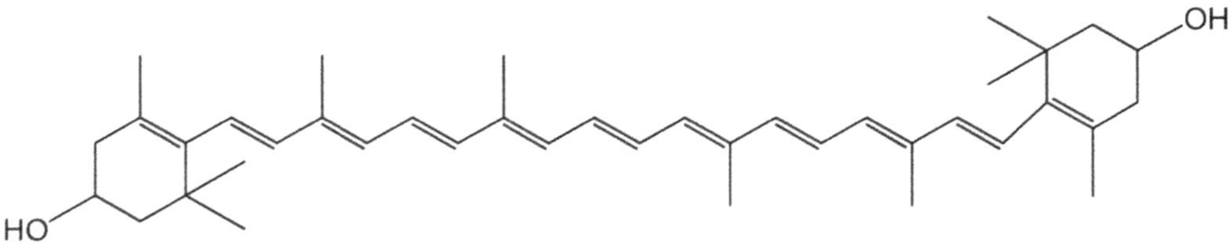

Zeaxanthin

Carotenoids has two major roles in plants; they absorb light energy required for photosynthesis and provides photoprotection by providing non photochemical quenching.

Therapeutic Uses

- Carotenoids acts as an antioxidant.
- Carotenoids have shown strong anti-inflammatory activity.
- Carotenoids are used as an anticancer agent.

Probable Questions

Long answer questions

1. Explain any two-indole alkaloid containing drugs in detail.

2. Write short note on cardiac glycosides. Explain Digitalis as cardiotonic drug.

3. What are volatile oils? Explain any two volatile oil containing drugs in detail.

Short answer questions

1. Write short note on carotenoids.

2. Write short note on chemistry of senna.

3. Explain the chemistry of dioscorea.

4. Write short note on aloe.

5. Write short note on phenylpropanoids containing drugs.

6. Explain in detail about the chemistry of vinca.

7. Explain Catechu in detail.

Very short answer questions

1. Write Biological source, chemical constituents, and therapeutic uses of ginger.

2. Write Biological source, chemical constituents, and therapeutic uses of artemisia.

3. Write Biological source, chemical constituents, and therapeutic uses of benzoin.

4. Write Biological source, chemical constituents, and therapeutic uses of Liquorice.

5. Write chemical test for tropane alkaloids.

6. Write chemical tests for anthraquinone alkaloids.

7. Write chemical test for cardiac glycoside.

8. Write short note on taxus.

9. Explain gentian drug in brief.

10. Explain in brief about deadly night shed leaf.

Unit III

Isolation, Identification and Analysis of Phytoconstituents

PCI Syllabus

Terpenoids: Menthol, Citral and Artemisinin; Glycosides: Glycyrrhetinic acid and Rutin; Alkaloids: Atropine, Quinine, Reserpine and Caffeine; Resins: Podophyllotoxin, Curcumin.

Book Chapter Contents

- Terpenoids
    - Introduction
    - Menthol
    - Citral
    - Artemisinin
- Glycosides
    - Introduction
    - Glycyrrhetinic Acid
    - Rutin
- Alkaloids
    - Introduction
    - Atropine
    - Quinine
    - Reserpine
    - Caffeine
- Resins
    - Introduction
    - Podophyllotoxins
    - Curcumin

Introduction

Crude drugs are usually complex mixtures containing thousands of different chemical constituents known as phytoconstituents. The extraction, isolation and determination of the therapeutically active components in medicinal plant can help us to study their pharmacological, pharmacokinetic and toxicological mechanisms. By using different extraction techniques, the phytoconstituents are extracted in suitable solvent. From the extract the desired phytoconstituent is isolated and then estimated for its purity. The extraction is a technique which helps us to separate the desired compounds from a mixture while the isolation is the technique to isolate and purify the only pure compound from the extracted compounds. The presence of other plant constituents (e.g. proteins, fats, sugars and tannins) in a crude extract makes the isolation of active constituents extremely difficult and powerful separation techniques with high efficiency and sensitivity are required. The increasing use of plant products has raised need for adequate methods and standards to ensure quality, safety and efficacy of these drugs and their preparations. The recent trends in herbal drug industry is focusing on the active phytoconstituents which are responsible for the therapeutic activity for better and specific effect at specific site. The commercially important phytoconstituents from alkaloids, glycosides, terpenoids and resins are discussed with respect to their isolation and identification techniques in this chapter.

Terpenoids

The terpenoids are also called as isoprenoids are a large and diverse class of naturally occurring organic compounds derived from basic structural unit known as terpenes. Terpenes are simple hydrocarbons, while terpenoids are modified class of terpenes with different functional groups and oxidized methyl group added or removed at different positions. Terpenes belong to the biggest class of secondary metabolites and basically consist of five carbon isoprene (C_5H_8) units which are assembled to each other (many isoprene units) by thousands of ways. Depending upon number of isoprene units terpenes are classified as Hemiterpene (Isoprene- C_5H_8), Monoterpenes ($C_{10}H_{16}$), Sesquiterpenes ($C_{15}H_{24}$), Diterpenes ($C_{20}H_{32}$), Triterpenes ($C_{30}H_{48}$), Tetraterpenes ($C_{40}H_{64}$) and polyterpenes (C_5H_8)$_n$.

Physical and chemical properties of terpenoids

- Terpenoids are colorless
- These are aromatic and volatile in nature
- All terpenoids are insoluble in water but are soluble in organic solvents
- Most of the terpenoids are optically active
- Terpenoids are either open chain structures or cyclic unsaturated compounds having one or more double bonds
- They undergo addition reaction with hydrogen, acids, alcohol or hydrogen
- Terpenoids also undergo polymerization and dehydrogenation reactions

- Terpenoids easily gets oxidized
- On thermal decomposition it gives isoprene as one product.

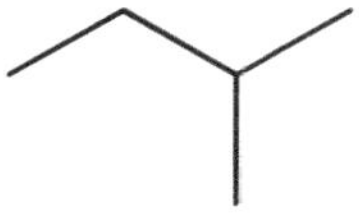

C_5 Hemiterpene (1 isoprene unit)

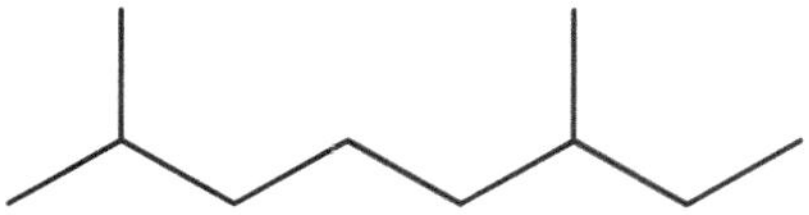

C_{10} Monoterpene (2 isoprene unit)

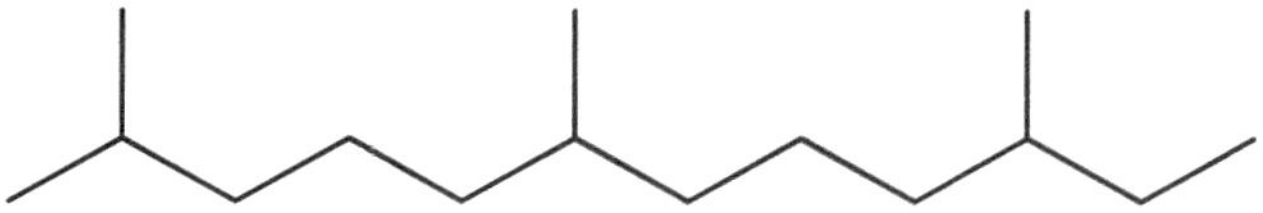

C_{15} Sesquiterpene (3 isoprene unit)

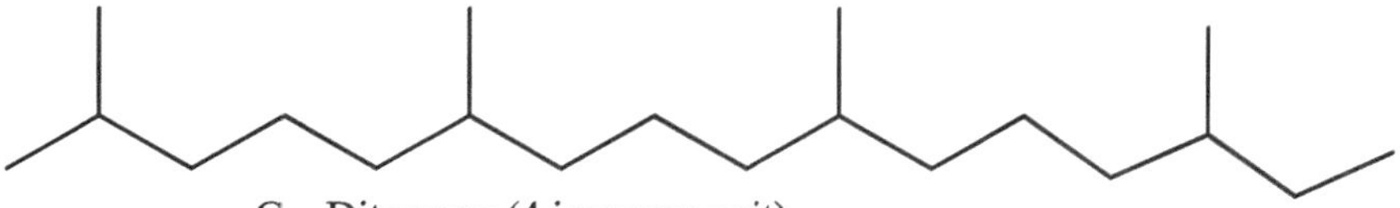

C_{20} Diterpene (4 isoprene unit)

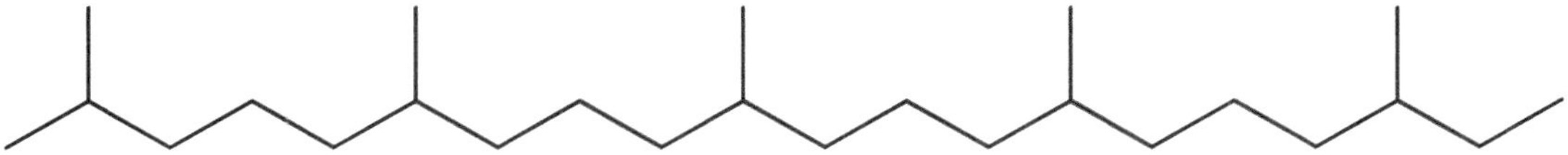

C_{25} Sesterpene (5 isoprene unit)

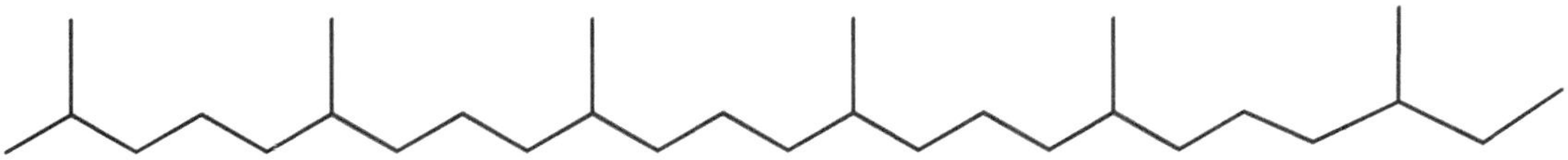

C_{30} triterpene (6 isoprene unit)

Examples of phytoconstituents from terpenoids

Menthol

Menthol is a monocyclic monoterpene alcohol obtained from various types of mint oils or peppermint. The sources of mint oil include black peppermint. *Mentha piperita*; *M. arvensis*, *M. Canadensis* and other Mentha species from family Lamiaceae. Peppermint contains about 1–3% of volatile oil and volatile oil contains not less than 45% of menthol. Along with menthol the oil contains (+) neomenthol, (+) isomenthol, menthone, menthofuran, menthyl acetate and cineol. The menthol obtained from the natural sources is Levorotatory (l-menthol) or racemic (dl-menthol). Menthol can be synthetically prepared by hydrogenation of thymol. Menthol provides a cooling sensation when applied to the skin or other tissues therefore used in food industry, in oral hygiene products, in therapeutic preparations to treat minor sore throat pain, or mouth irritation caused by a canker sore. Menthol is also used in many topical preparations for its analgesic and counter irritant properties.

Isolation of Menthol

1. The first step in the isolation of menthol is separation of peppermint oil by hydro distillation or steam distillation of whole plant above ground just before flowering.

2. The obtained oil is then passed through anhydrous sodium sulphate to make it moisture free.

3. This oil is then cooled below -22 °C in tightly closed container for about 7-8 days. The crystals of menthol crystallize out from the oil which are separated by filtration. The crystals of menthol are squeezed between filter paper to remove adhering oil and finally recovered by recrystallization.

4. Still the filtrate contains some amount of menthol along with menthone and other terpenes. To remove menthone, the filtrate is treated with boric acid followed by boiling for further 3 hours. The released menthone is removed by distillation.

5. The filtrate now contains borate of menthol which is saponified with alcoholic potassium hydroxide by heating under reflux for about 1 hour.

6. The obtained solution is allowed to cool where remaining menthol crystals separates out.

7. Crystals obtained by direct cooling and by saponification are mixed and dried properly.

Identification Tests for Menthol

- Melting point: 41–44 °C.

- On heating the crystals of menthol in watch glass on boiling water bath, the entire crystals evaporate without leaving any residue.

- Mix the small quantity of menthol with equal volume of thymol/ camphor in a test tube. Liquification of the contents in the test tube indicates the presence of menthol.

- Dissolve 10 mg of menthol crystals in 4 drops of conc. sulphuric acid. To this add few drops of vanillin sulphuric acid reagent, solution shows orange yellow coloration that changes to violet after adding few drops of water.

- Dissolve few crystals of menthol in glacial acetic acid and add 4 ml mixture (3 ml of sulphuric acid and 1 ml of nitric acid). It fails to produce either green or bluish green coloration (thymol gives green coloration)

Analysis/Estimation of Menthol

A variety of methods are available for the estimation of menthol viz. titrimetric method, TLC, RP-HPLC, gas chromatography etc.

A. Titrimetric Method

- Weigh accurately 2 gm of Menthol and add 20 ml of mixture of dehydrated pyridine and acetic anhydride (8:1) in a flask.

- Connect the reflux condenser and heat on a water bath for two hours.

- Cool the solution and remove the condenser.

- Wash the condenser with 20 ml of water and titrate the content of the flask with 1M alcoholic sodium hydroxide solution using phenolphthalein as an indicator. Note down the reading as 'a' ml.

- Perform blank determination and note down reading as 'b' ml.

- (b-a) gives the number of ml of titrant equivalent to the acetic acid used up for the acetylation of menthol.

- Determine the percentage of free menthol from the equivalent factor of 1M alcoholic sodium hydroxide 156.27 mg.

B. Thin Layer Chromatography of Menthol

Dissolve about 1 mg of menthol in about 1 ml of methanol. Apply the spot on the silica gel-GF_{254} plate and elute it in pure chloroform. Spray the dried plates with 1% vanillin sulphuric acid reagent and heat the plate at 110 °C for 10 min. Menthol *Rf* value is 0.48–0.62 in normal chamber saturation at 24 °C.

Citral

Citral occurs abundantly in lemon grass oil (75 to 80%) obtained by steam distillation of *Cymbopogon citratus* / *Cymbopogon flexosus* from Graminae family. It is also found to limited extent in the oil of verbena, lemon, lime, orange, ginger root and several citrus species. Citral is a mixture of two geometric isomers called Geranial and Neral.

Geranial
(*trans*)

Neral
(*cis*)

Isolaion of Citral

1. The lemongrass oil is thoroughly shaken with 5% (w/v) sodium bisulphite solution for about 25 to 30 minutes.

2. Separate the resulting crystalline adduct on a Buchner funnel, and subsequently wash it with solvent ether or ethanol to remove the impurities.

3. Decompose the sodium bisulphite adduct with dilute sodium hydroxide solution carefully to obtain crude citral.

4. Finally, the pure citral is obtained by distilling the crude citral cautiously under reduced pressure.

5. ***Separation of Geranial and Neral:*** Sodium bisulphate complex of Geranial is sparingly soluble while sodium bisulphate complex of Neral is readily soluble in water. This property can be used to separate Geranial and Neral. Similarly, if citral (mixture of Geranial and Neral) is shaken with alkaline cyanoacetic acid solution for a short time, geranial reacts with this acid faster to form Geranial cyanoacetic anhydride.

Identification Tests for Citral

- As citral consist of two ethylenic and one aldehydic linkage; it is very sensitive to oxidizing agents (even air exposure) and gives linalool which is having intense yellow color.

- Geranial on treatment with Tollen's reagent produces geranic acid.

- Hydrogenation of geranial with sodium amalgum in slightly acidic solution gives rise to citronellal and citronellol.

- Geranial when treated with potassium bisulphite it gets converted to *para –cymene.*

Estimation of Citral

A. **By Colorimetry:** The citral content of lemongrass oil can be estimated by the coloring agent - that of Ehrlich Miller. This coloring agent has been found to give better results and development of color takes place rapidly and remain quite stable for a long time. The coloring agent is prepared according to Ehrlich Miller and consist of the following solutions.

1. 5% *p*-dimethylaminobenzaldehyde solution in acetic acid.

2. 10% phosphoric acid solution in acetic acid.

One ml each of the above solutions are added to different amounts of citral in acetic acid, whereby a marked color change from blue to pink can be observed. The percentage absorbance and extinction of the colored citral is then measured using colorimeter and calibration graphs are plotted. The amount of citral in solutions can be compared with that of known strength and thus the percentage of citral can be determined.

B. HPTLC method

Stationary Phase: 20 cm × 10 cm aluminum foil-backed HPTLC plates coated with 200-μm layers of silica gel $60F_{254.}$

Mobile Phase: Linear ascending development of the plates is generally performed by using toluene–ethyl acetate 8.5:1.5 (v/v) as binary mobile phase.

Visualization of plates: Plates are visualized by spraying with vanillin–sulfuric acid reagent; prepared by dissolving 0.5 g vanillin in 85:10:5 (v/v) methanol–glacial acetic acid–sulfuric acid mixture. Well defined spots were obtained when the chamber was saturated with mobile phase for 30 min at 25 ± 2°C at *Rf* 0.55 ± 0.03 and 0.34 ± 0.05 for trans and cis-citral, respectively.

Densitometric method: Densitometric scanning, at 595 nm is done with a CAMAG TLC Scanner III in absorbance mode. Different concentrations of both cis and trans citral spotted on a plate. Toluene–ethyl acetate 8.5:1.5 (v/v) gives sharp, compact, and well defined peaks at *Rf* 0.55 ± 0.03 and 0.34 ± 0.05 for trans and cis-citral, respectively.

C. By using Gas liquid Chromatography: Citral can be estimated by gas liquid chromatography coupled with a non-polar capillary column using Flame Ionization Detector.

Artemisinin

Artemisinin is an antimalarial drug obtained from Chinese traditional herb *Artemisia annua* (family- Astreaceae). The parasite responsible for malarial infection is *plasmodium falciparum*. The first effective antimalarial agent to treat this infection is quinine and its derivatives like chloroquine, mefloquine etc. But malarial parasite developed resistance to these drugs. Hence the naturally obtained artemisinin and its semisynthetic derivatives are considered as most effective for the treatment of malaria by Artemisinin combination therapy (ACT's) or monotherapy. Artemisinin was discovered by a Chinese scientist Tu Youyou in 1972. It is a sesquiterpene lactone endoperoxide containing a rare peroxide linkage which is essential for activity. Artemisinin also showed anticancer activity in preclinical studies. It is soluble in organic solvents and insoluble in water.

Artemisinin

Isolation of Artemisinin

1. Powder the dried leaves of *Artemisia annua* and extract with methanol using kinetic maceration technique. The kinetic maceration can be repeated many times till the methanol becomes colorless.

2. Pool the methanol extracts together and reduce the volume to 100 ml under vacuum at 40 °C.

3. Partition the methanol extract with hexane several times till the hexane layer become colorless.

4. Now two fractions are available; methanolic and hexane fraction.

5. Add little amount of water to the methanol extract to make it hydroalcoholic. Partition this hydroalcoholic extract with ethyl acetate. The process is repeated several times till the ethyl acetate layer is colorless.

6. Separate two fractions; ethyl acetate fraction is semipolar and hydroalcoholic fraction is polar fraction.

7. Reduce both fractions under vacuum at 40 °C separately.

8. The most viscous extract contains artemisinin. The extract is fractionated by using column chromatography where silica gel 60 is used as stationary phase and mixture of ethyl acetate: hexane as mobile phase with increasing polarity (gradient elution technique). Each separated fraction in column is collected separately and identified for the presence of artemisinin.

9. The identification is carried out by using TLC method where Silica gel 60 is used as stationary phase and Ethyl acetate: Hexane as mobile phase.

10. The fractions showing presence of Artemisinin is then used for preparative TLC to obtain artemisinin.

Identification test for artemisinin: The presence of artemisinin is checked by TLC method by using mobile phase n- hexane: Ethyl Acetate (75:25, v/v) and derivatizing with anisaldehyde sulphuric acid reagent. Artemisinin get separated at *Rf* 0.28.

Estimation/ Analysis of Artemisinin

A. Estimation by HPLC: A series of solutions of known concentrations of artemisinin and predetermined concentration of *A. annua* extract samples are prepared for the analysis of artemisinin in plant extract by reverse phase liquid chromatography. C_{18} column is used as stationary phase while formic acid (% 0.2 v/v): acetonitrile (50:50) is used as mobile phase. The isocratic elution technique is chosen to achieve maximum separation and sensitivity by maintaining flow rate 1.0 ml/min. The samples were detected at 254 nm using photodiode array detector. Results of artemisinin quantities in Artemisia samples were expressed as the mean of three determinations by using calibration curve.

B. Estimation by HPTLC: The known concentration of hexane extract of *A. annua* is used as test solution while standard artemisinin of known purity and known concentration dissolved in hexane is used as standard solution. The TLC plate is developed using mobile phase n- Hexane: Ethyl Acetate (75:25, v/v) in a saturated chamber. After development plate is derivatized with anisaldehyde- sulphuric acid reagent followed by heating at 110 °C for 10 min. The presence of pink color spot at *Rf* 0.28 confirms the presence of artemisinin. Similarly, the plate is scanned using HPTLC densitometer at 540 nm. By using calibration curve, the quantity of the artemisinin in sample is calculated.

Glycosides

Glycosides are the compounds that yields one or more sugar moieties on hydrolysis. The glycoside is a generic term for natural product that is chemically bound to a sugar. "Glycosides may be defined as the organic compounds from plant or animal origin which on enzymatic/ acid hydrolysis yields one or more sugar moieties along with nonsugar moieties". Sugar portion is known as **Glycone** and non sugar portion as **Aglycone**. The linkage between glycone and aglycone is called as **Glycosidic linkage**.

General properties of glycosides:

- Glycosides are crystalline, amorphous substance.
- Glycosides are easily hydrolyzed by water, mineral acids and enzymes.
- Glycosides are optically active, generally Levo rotatory.
- They do not reduce Fehling's solution until they are hydrolyzed.
- Though glycoside contains sugar, the physical, chemical and therapeutic properties are attributed to aglycone part. The glycone portion facilitates absorption of glycosides and helps in transportation of aglycone part to reach the site of action.
- Glycosides are soluble in water and dilute alcohol except resin glycosides and insoluble in organic solvents. Aglycone part is soluble in organic solvents.

Glycyrrhetinic Acid

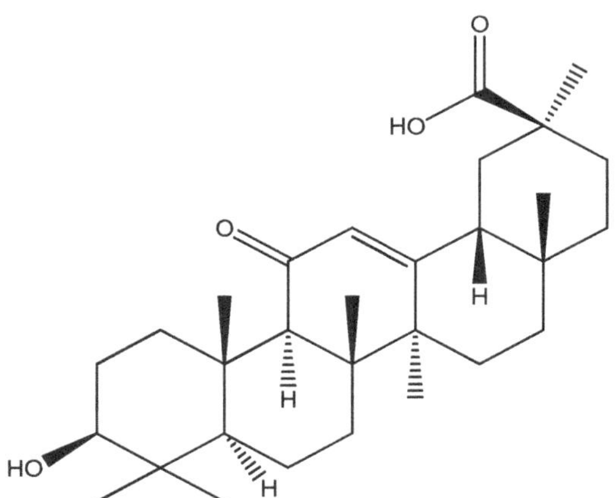

Glycyrrhetinic acid

Glycyrrhetinic acid is a pentacyclic triterpenoid aglycone of β-amyrin type obtained from the plant roots and rhizomes of Liquorice (*Glycerrhyza glabra*; family- Leguminosae). It is also known as Glycyrrhetic acid or Enoxolone. It is a hydrolysis product of Glycyrrhizin – a major glycoside present in liquorice. It is widely used in the treatment of peptic ulcer and as an expectorant. It is also used as flavoring agent in pharmaceuticals and also to mask the taste of bitter drugs like aloe and quinine. Glycyrrhetinic acid exerts mineralocorticoid activity and hence used in treatment of inflammations, rheumatoid arthritis and Addison's disease.

Isolation of Glycyrrhetinic acid

Method 1

1. Take about 20g of powdered drug, add 50 ml of acetone and 2ml of dilute nitric acid to it. Mix thoroughly and macerate for about 2 h with occasional shaking.

2. Filter the contents, extract again with small amount of acetone by heating on a boiling water bath. Filter and combine the filtrates, concentrate the filtrate under vaccum.

3. To the acetone extract add sufficient quantity of dilute ammonia solution; so as to precipitate ammonium glycerrhizinate.

4. Separate the precipitate by filtration followed by washing with 5-10 ml of acetone.

5. Dry the product and weigh to find out the yield. Generally,4-5% w/w yield is expected.

Method 2

1. Extract the accurately weighed quantity of the liquorice powder with chloroform in Soxhlet apparatus for about 6 h.

2. Filter the content of the flask and discard the filtrate.

3. Extract the marc with 0.5 M sulphuric acid for 2-3 h.

4. Filter the content of the flask

5. Extract the filtrate in separating funnel with 25 ml of chloroform. Repeat the process three times.

6. Combine the chloroform extracts and evaporate to dryness. Residue of glycyrrhetinic acid is formed.

Identification tests for Glycyrrhetinic Acid:

Libermann Test: Mix 2ml of test solution with 2 ml of acetic anhydride, boil and add 0.5 ml of sulphuric acid. Appearance of blue colour indicates the presence of glycyrrhetinic acid.

Estimation of Glycyrrhetinic Acid

By using TLC- densitometry

Stationary phase: Kieselghar 60 HF coated on TLC plate

Mobile phase: n-butanol: Acetic acid: water (7:1:2)

Visualizing agent: 1% cerric sulphate in 10% sulphuric acid followed by heating at 105°C for 5 min.

Standard solution preparation: A known concentration of glycyrrhetinic acid (0.5 to 2 mg/ml) in ethanol.

Sample solution: Reflux 1gm of sample with 50 ml of 50% ethanol cool and filter. Reflux the marc with 50 ml of 50% ethanol. Evaporate and dissolve the residues in 50% ethanol (10 ml).

Development of chromatograms: Around 13-14 cm

Visualization of spots: Generally the spots are visualized and scanned in densitometer. The area of spots corresponding to glycyrrhetinic acid is integrated and then calculated the percentage of it in the sample.

Rutin

Rutin is obtained from the buck wheat which comprises of dried riped fruits of *Fagopyrum esculentum*, family- Polygonaceae. The other sources of Rutin are; *Ruta graveolense* (family- Rutaceae), fresh leaves of tobacco plant *Nicotiana tobacum*; family –Solanaceae. The highest yield of glycoside is obtained from buckwheat leaves and flowers as soon as the plant attains the blossom stage, after the maturation the glycoside content decreases. Rutin is insoluble in water, ether, petroleum ether and chloroform. It is soluble in ethanol and acetone. Rutin is used to decrease the capillary fragility, reduces capillary permeability by tissue injury. It is used in treatment of retinal hemorrhages.

Rutin

Isolation of Rutin

1. The dried and ground plant material (150 g) is extracted with two successive quantities of 80% ethanol (2× 200ml).
2. The hydroalcoholic extract is filtered and reduced to 50-60 ml.
3. The extract is partitioned with ether in a separating funnel.
4. Repeat the partitioning and discard the ether layer.
5. Reduce the aqueous extract to 10 ml.
6. Cool below 5 °C overnight, rutin crystals separate outs. Filter the solution.
7. The crude rutin obtained by this way subjected to column chromatography for further purification.

Identification tests for Rutin

- Rutin with basic lead acetate gives distinct yellow color.
- Rutin treated with ferric chloride solution shows greenish brown color.

Estimation of Rutin

By spectrophotometry

Sample solution preparation: Dissolve 0.5 mg of sample in 50 ml of methanol and filter. Take 2 ml of filtrate in a 50 ml volumetric flask add 2 ml of double distilled water and 5 ml of ammoinum molybdate. Adjust the volume up to the mark with water.

Standard solution preparation: Dissolve 0.5 mg of standard in 50 ml of methanol and filter. Further follow the procedure as per sample solution preparation.

Measure the absorbance of standard and sample solution at 360 nm. Percentage of rutin can be calculated by using the following formula

$$\% \text{ of Rutin} = \frac{A_{sample} \times C \times 50 \times 100}{A_{standard} \times W \times 2}$$

A sample = Absorbance of sample at 360nm

A standard = Absorbance of standard at 360nm

C = concentration of standard solution (g/ml)

W = weight of the sample

Alkaloids

Alkaloids are the organic products of natural or synthetic origin which are basic in nature and contains one or more nitrogen atoms, normally of heterocyclic nature and possesses specific physiological action on human or animal body when used even in small quantities.

Based on the origin and position of nitrogen, alkaloids are categorized as follows.

True alkaloids: These are derived from amino acid and contains nitrogen inside the heterocyclic ring. Example- Atropine

Proto alkaloid: These are derived from amino acids but do not contain nitrogen in heterocyclic ring. Example- Ephedrine

Pseudo alkaloids: These are not derived from amino acids but have nitrogen inside the heterocyclic ring. They may not show many typical characters of alkaloids but give standard qualitative tests of alkaloids positive. Example- Conesine.

General Properties of alkaloids:

- Generally, alkaloids are colorless crystalline solids with sharp melting point.

- Some are amorphous in nature while conine, nicotine are liquid in nature.

- Most alkaloids are also chiral molecules. This results in isomers that have different chemical properties i.e. one isomer may have a physiological function while the other does not.

- Free bases of alkaloids are soluble in organic solvents but insoluble in water while the salts of most alkaloids are soluble in water.

- In nature, alkaloids exists either in free state, as amine or as a salt with acid or alkaloid N-oxides.

General chemical tests for Alkaloids

Mayer's Test: Drug solution + few drops of Mayer's reagent (potassium mercuric iodide), formation of creamy-white precipitate.

Wagner's Test: Drug solution + few drops of Wagner's reagent (dilute Iodine solution), formation of reddish-brown precipitate.

Dragendorff's Test: Drug solution + Dragendroff's reagent (Potassium bismuth Iodide), formation of Orange red color.

Hager's Test: Drug solution + few drops of Hager's reagent (Saturated aqueous solution of Picric acid), formation of crystalline yellow precipitate.

Tannic Acid Test: Drug solution + few drops of tannic acid solution, formation of buff colored precipitate.

General Extraction methods

Method A

The powdered material that contains alkaloidal salts is moistened with alkaline substances like sodium bicarbonate, ammonia, calcium hydroxide, etc., which combines with acids, tannins and other phenolic substances and sets free the alkaloids bases. Extraction is then carried out with organic solvents such as ether or petroleum spirit. The concentrated organic liquid is then shaken with aqueous acid and allowed to separate. Alkaloid salts will be present in aqueous liquid, while many impurities remain behind in the organic liquid.

Method B

The collected powdered material is extracted with water or aqueous alcohol containing dilute acid. Chloroform or other organic solvents are added and shaken to remove the pigments and other unwanted materials. The free alkaloids are then precipitated by the addition of excess alkalis like, sodium bicarbonate or ammonia and separated by filtration or by extraction with organic solvents. Volatile liquid alkaloids (nicotine and coniine) are isolated by distillation. The powdered material that contains alkaloids is extracted with water and the aqueous extract is made alkaline with sodium carbonate or ammonia and the alkaloid is distilled off in steam. This could be collected and purified.

Atropine

Atropine is a tropane alkaloid obtained from dried leaves of *Atropa belladonna* (European belladonna) or *Atropa accuminata* (Indian belladona), family- Solanaceae. It is commonly known as belladonna or deadly nightshade leaf.

Atropine is used as a mydriatic to dilate pupil of the eye, and also used to reduce the secretions like saliva, tears, sweat and gastric juices. It is used as antidote in pilocarpine poisoning. It is also administered intravenously for the treatment of bradycardia. Atropine is very soluble in ethanol; slightly soluble in chloroform.

Isolation of Atropine

1. The drug material in powdered form is first extracted with ethanol.

2. Filter and evaporate the solvent to yield syrupy extract. Treat the extract with dilute hydrochloric acid in order to form alkaloidal salt, and resinous matter will get precipitate out.

3. Filter the solution; resinous matter retained on the filter paper.

4. The acidic solution partitioned with petroleum ether/ chloroform in a separating funnel.

5. The chloroform/ petroleum ether layer is collected and removed by distillation to get the crude alkaloidal mixture which is further treated with oxalic acid.

6. The oxalates of atropine and hyoscyamine are separated by fractional crystallization from acetone and ether which gives the atropine oxalates crystals.

Identification Tests

Vithali Morin Test: To the extract add fuming nitric acid and evaporate to dryness on water bath. To the nitrated residue add methanolic potassium hydroxide solution, appearance of deep purple color indicates the presence of tropane alkaloid.

Rathenasinkam's test: Heat 0.5 mg of atropine with nitric acid for 10 min and add 30 ml of water. Extract the solution with chloroform. Allow it to separate in separating funnel. Discard chloroform layer. To the aqueous layer add few drops of ammonia and again extract with chloroform. Evaporate the chloroform layer; to the residue add acetone and few drops of 10% sodium hydroxide. Appearance of bluish purple color indicates the presence of atropine.

Estimation of Atropine

A. Assay of atropine sulphate by titrimetric method

The atropine content as atropine sulphate is determined by titrimetric method. The accurately weighed quantity of test solution i.e. sulphate salt dissolved in 50 ml of glacial acetic acid and titrated with 0.1 N perchloric acid and endpoint is determined by potentiometry.

The blank determination is also carried out and the amount of atropine sulphate is calculated by using the factor;

Each ml of 0.1 N perchloric acid is equivalent to 0.06770 gm of atropine sulphate.

B. By TLC

Standard solution: 1% solution of atropine is added to 2N acetic acid

Stationary phase: Silica gel G

Mobile phase: Strong ammonia solution: methanol (1.5: 100)

Derivatizing agent: Dragendorff's reagent

Rf value: 0.18

Quinine

Quinine is obtained from bark of different species of cinchona viz. *Cinchona officinalis, C.calisaya, C. ledgeriana, C. succirubra* (family - Rubiaceae). It is a quinoline type of alkaloid. Cinchona consists of quinine, quinindine, cinchonine and cinchonidine. Quinine and quinidine are stereoisomers of each other and they form many salts, but therapeutically sulphates are used commonly.

The total alkaloid content varies with different species from 5 to 10 %. *C.ledgiarana* contains around 6-10 % of total alkaloids wherein 75% is quinine. Quinine is used as an antimalarial drug.

Quinine

Isolation of quinine

1. Thoroughly mix finely powdered cinchona bark with sufficient quantity of calcium hydroxide solution and convert it to paste by mixing 5% of sodium hydroxide solution.

2. Extract the paste with benzene in Soxhlet extractor for 6 h.

3. Transfer the resultant extract into the separating funnel and extract several times with warm dilute sulphuric acid for complete extraction of alkaloids.

4. The pH of acid layer is adjusted to about 6.5 by the addition of sodium hydroxide solution.

5. Allow the resultant mixture to cool and then centrifuge it for the separation of crystals of quinine sulphate.

6. Purify the quinine sulphate obtained by recrystallization from hot water.

7. Dissolve quinine sulphate crystals in warm dilute sulphuric acid; to this add dilute ammonia solution till solution becomes alkaline.

8. Quinine precipitate out as amorphous crystals, filter it and wash with water to remove sodium, ammonium salts.

Identification Tests for Quinine

- **Thalleoquin test**

  To the small quantity of dilute acidic solution of quinine in test tube add few ml of bromine water with gentle shaking. After addition of dilute ammonia solution, the formation of emerald green color which turns to blue after neutralization indicates the presence of quinine.

- To the little quantity of quinine in test tube add little quantity of glacial acetic acid. After heating the mixture in a test tube, formation of purple vapors at the upper part indicates the presence of quinine.

Estimation of quinine

By TLC

Stationary Phase: Silica gel G coated TLC plates

Mobile phase: Chloroform: methanol: ammonia (60:10:1)

Preparation of standard quinine solution: 1 mg/ml solution of standard quinine is prepared by dissolving 1 mg of quinine in 1 ml of chloroform.

Preparation of sample solution: 1mg/ ml solution of reduced cinchona extract is prepared in chloroform.

Both the sample and standard solution are applied on TLC plate and allow to develop in previously saturated development chamber.

Rf value of quinine is 0.6.

Reserpine

Reserpine is an indole alkaloid obtained from the roots of plant *Rauwolfia serpentina* (family-Apocyanaceae). Reserpine is a commonly used drug for the treatment of high blood pressure. It is a adrenergic blocking agent and hence used as antihypertensive agent to treat mild to moderate hypertension. Reserpine is lipid soluble and can cross blood brain barrier and hence it is also used as a tranquillizer.

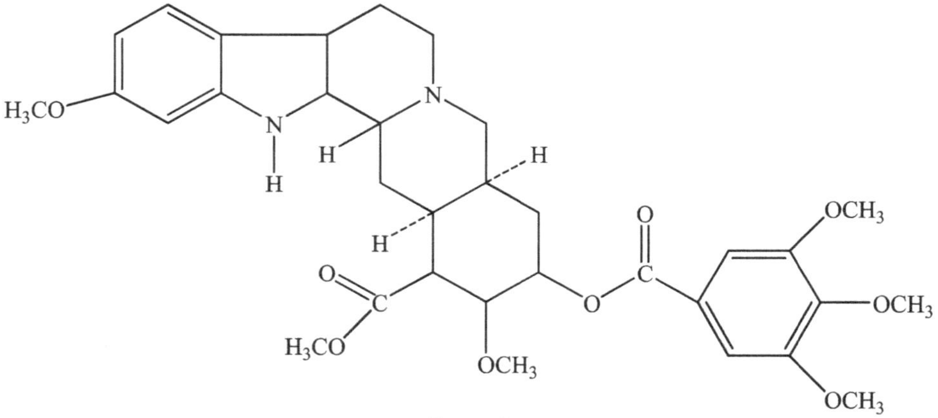

Reserpine

Isolation of Reserpine

1. Extract the Rauwolfia root powder exhaustively with 90% alcohol by maceration or percolation.
2. Concentrate the alcoholic extract and dry under reduced pressure below 60°C to yield rauwolfia dry extract containing about 4% of total alkaloids.
3. Rauwolfia dry extract is extracted further with proportions of ether–chloroform–90% alcohol (20:8:2.5).
4. To the extract obtained, add little dilute ammonia with intermittent shaking. Alkaloid is converted to water-insoluble base.
5. Add water and allow the drug to settle after few vigorous shakings.
6. Fitter off the solution and extract the residue with 4 volumes of 0.5 N H_2SO_4 in separating funnel.

7. Combine the total acid extract which contains the alkaloidal salt.

8. The extract is filtered, made alkaline with dilute ammonia to liberate alkaloid.

9. Finally, it is extracted with chloroform.

10. The total chloroform extract is filtered; chloroform is removed by distillation and the total alkaloidal extract is dried under vacuum to yield total rauwolfia alkaloids.

11. Total rauwolfia alkaloid consists of the mixture of over 30 different components.

12. Subject it to column chromatographic fractionation for the separation of reserpine.

Identification tests for Reserpine: To the drug extract add solution of vanillin in acetic acid; formation of violet red color indicates the presence of reserpine.

Estimation of Reserpine

Melting point: 270 °C

By Chromatographic Study (TLC)

Stationary phase: Silica gel-G plates

Mobile phase: chloroform–acetone–diethylamine (50:40:30)

Sample and test solution preparation: Dissolve 1 mg of rauwolfia alkaloidal extract or pure reserpine in 1 ml of methanol.

Apply the spots over the TLC plate and allow to run.

Note down the distance travelled by solute and solvent and calculate *Rf* value.

The *Rf* value was found to be 0.72

Caffeine

Caffeine is a methylated xanthene alkaloid derivative obtained from the tea plant (*Thea sinensis*; family- Theaceae) and coffee beans (*Caffea arabica*; family- Rubiaceae). The caffeine percentage in coffee beans found around 1-2% while in tea leave 1-5 %.

Caffeine can be isolated from cocoa seeds (*Theobroma cacao*; family Sterculiaceae), Kola seeds (*Cola acuminate*; family- Sterculiaceae).

Caffeine acts as a CNS stimulant, mild diuretic and prescribed for the treatment of migraine with ergotamine and with aspirin for analgesic effect.

Caffeine

Generally isolation of caffeine is done by using tea leaves powder. Other than alkaloids tea leaves contain cellulose, tannins and chlorophyll. Caffeine is highly soluble in dichloromethane and also soluble in hot water.

Isolation of Caffeine

1. Take about 30 gm of tea leaves and to this 250 ml of water. Add 5 gm of sodium carbonate in the solution to remove the tannins.

2. Boil the solution for 10 min.

3. Filter the solution while hot.

4. Extract the marc with 100 ml of water.

5. Combine the water extracts and allow to cool.

6. Partition the water extract with 25 ml of dichloromethane in a separating funnel.

7. Collect the dichloromethane layer.

8. Repeat the process again 2 times to ensure complete extraction and combine the extracts.

9. Filter the dichloromethane extract through the bed of anhydrous sodium carbonate packed on glass funnel with cotton wool to remove any moisture present.

10. Evaporate dichloromethane, silky crystals of caffeine can be observed which can be recrystallized by hot ethanol.

Identification tests for Caffeine

- ***Murexide test***: Caffeine and other purine alkaloids, gives murexide color reaction. Take Caffeine in a petridish, add hydrochloric acid and potassium chlorate, evaporate to dryness. Expose the residue to dilute ammonia solution. Formation of purple color indicates the presence of caffeine. In addition of fixed alkali the purple color disappears.

- With tannic acid solution Caffeine produces white precipitate.

Estimation of Caffeine

By Chromatographic Study (TLC)

Stationary phase: Silica gel G coated TLC plate

Mobile phase: Ethyl acetate: methanol: acetic acid (80:10:10)

Sample and standard solution preparation: 1mg /ml solution of both standard caffeine and tea leaves extract is prepared in methanol.

The standard and sample solutions are spotted on TLC plates and kept in already saturated chamber for development. After development plate is dried and sprayed with Dragendorffs reagent.

Rf value for caffeine is 0.41

Resins

Resins are defined as the complex amorphous product of more or less solid characteristics which on heating first get softened and then melt. Resins are produced and stored in the schizogenous or schizolysigenous glands or cavities of the plants. Isolated resin products available in market are more or less solid, hard, transparent, or translucent materials. Resins are mixture of organic compounds like volatile oils, oxygenated products of terpenes and carboxylic acids. Resins are insoluble in most polar and nonpolar solvents like water and petroleum ether, respectively, but dissolve completely in alcohol, solvent ether, benzene, or chloroform.

Podophyllotoxin

Podophyllotoxin is a lignin derivative of podophyllin-a resinous matter obtained from dried roots and rhizomes of *Podophyllum peltatum* (American podophyllum) and *Podophyllum hexandrum* (Indian podophyllum); family-Berberidaceae. The resin should contain not less than 40 % of podophyllotoxin. Podophyllotoxin shows cytotoxic activity hence it is used for the treatment of venereal and other warts.

Podophyllotoxin is used as a precursor for semisynthetic anticancer drugs like etoposide and teniposide which is mainly used for the treatment of lung and testicular cancer. Podophyllum resin is a strong gastrointestinal irritant and acts as a drastic purgative.

Podophyllotoxin is insoluble in diethyl ether, slightly soluble in water, soluble in acetone, benzene and very soluble in ethanol and chloroform.

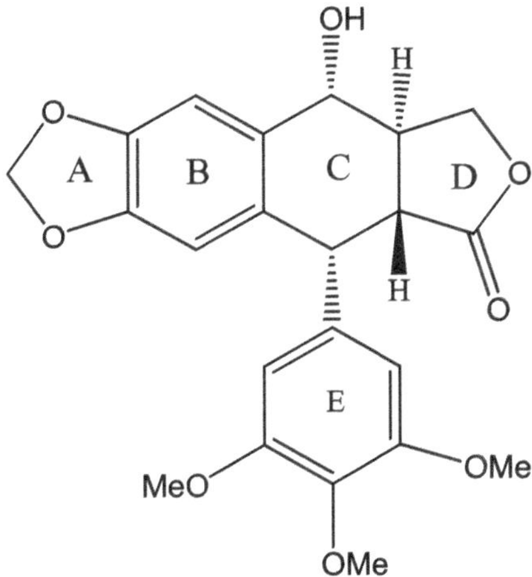

Podophyllotoxin

Isolation of Podophyllotoxin:

1. Extract the powdered podophyllum with methanol in soxhelet extractor.
2. Filter the extract and reduce the volume under reduced pressure to syrupy consistency.
3. To this add very dilute hydrochloric acid (10 ml diluted to 100 ml) and keep aside for 30 minutes.
4. Resinous matter precipitates, filter the solution and wash the resin several times with cold water.
5. After drying brown color precipitate of podophyllin is obtained.
6. Dissolve the residue in sufficient quantity of hot 90 % ethanol, filter and evaporate to dryness.
7. Re-crystallize the residue in benzene to yield podophyllotoxin.

Identification tests for Podophyllotoxin

- Podophyllotoxin when treated with 50% sulphuric acid shows violet blue coloration.
- When podophyllin treated with 90% alcohol followed by treatment with strong copper acetate solution ; formation of brown color precipitate.

Estimation of podophyllotoxin

By TLC:

Stationary phase: Silica gel G coated TLC plate

Mobile phase: Toulene: Ethyl acetate (5:7)

Sample and standard solution preparation: 1mg /ml solution of both standard podophyllotoxin and podophyllum extract is prepared in methanol.

The standard and sample solutions are spotted on TLC plates and kept in already saturated chamber for development. After development plate is dried and sprayed with sulphuric acid solution.

Rf value for podophyllotoxin is 0.39.

Curcumin

Curcumin is a bright yellow colored resin obtained from the fresh as well as dried rhizomes of turmeric i.e.*Curcuma longa* (family- Zingiberaceae). Turmeric is a traditional medicine in Ayurvedic, Unani and Chinese systems of medicines. Curcumin present in turmeric is a diarylheptanoid belonging to the group of curcuminoids. These curcuminoids are natural phenols and responsible for the yellow color of the turmeric. Curcumin is insoluble in water and ether; very soluble in ethanol and glacial acetic acid.

Curcumin is commonly used as a condiment. It is used as antiinflammatory, antiarthritic, stomachic, cholegaugge. It is also used in bronchitis and cough

Curcumin

Isolation of Curcumin

1. Extract the turmeric powder by using 95% of methanol in Soxhlet apparatus.
2. Filter the solution and evaporate the methanol till semisolid consistency is achieved.
3. Dissolve the semisolid extract in benzene followed by extraction with 0.1 % sodium hydroxide solution in separating funnel.

4. Collect the alkaline layer and acidify by addition with hydrochloric acid which will result in the formation of yellow colored precipitate.

5. Concentrate the extract by heating on a boiling water bath and simultaneously dissolve the precipitate in boiling water which results in formation of lumpy mass.

6. Filter the solution while hot and concentrate the filtrate to a very small volume and finally cool to get curcumin.

Identification tests for Curcumin: Curcumin when treated with acid, color changes to crimson red color. Curcumin when treated with alkali, color changes to red to violet color.

Estimation of Curcumin

By Chromatography study- TLC

Stationary phase: Silica gel G coated TLC plate

Mobile phase: Chloroform: Ethanol: Glacial acetic acid (94: 5: 1)

Sample and standard solution preparation: 1mg /ml solution of both standard curcumin and turmeric extract is prepared in methanol.

The standard and sample solutions are spotted on TLC plates and kept in already saturated chamber for development. After development plate is dried and observed under 366 nm.

Rf value for curcumin is 0.79.

Probable Questions

Long answer questions

1. Write in detail about the method of isolation and estimation of Caffeine.

2. Write short note on isolation of antimalarial drug.

3. What are glycosides? Explain in detail the isolation and estimation of rutin.

Short answer questions

1. Explain the simple method of isolation of indole alkaloid.

2. Write chemical structure and identification tests of Citral.

3. Explain different methods of isolation of Artemisinin.

4. Write short note on estimation of Reserpine.

Very short answer questions

1. Write structure of Atropine and Curcumin.

2. Write identification tests for Caffeine.

3. Write any two estimation methods of Podophyllotoxin.

4. Write specific chemical test for tropane alkaloids.

5. Write structure of Caffeine and Podophyllotoxin.

6. Write chemical test for Atropine.

Unit IV

Industrial Production, Estimation and Utilization of Phytoconstituents

PCI Syllabus

Forskolin, Sennoside, Artemisinin, Diosgenin, Digoxin, Atropine, Podophyllotoxin, Caffeine, Taxol, Vincristine and Vinblastine

Book Chapter Contents

- Introduction

Industrial Production, Estimation and Utilization of Following Phytoconstituents

- Forskolin
- Sennosides
- Artemisinin
- Diosgenin
- Digoxin
- Atropine
- Podophyllotoxin
- Caffeine
- Taxol
- Vincristine and Vinblastine

Introduction

Till now we have seen the methods of isolation and estimation of different phytoconstituents from herbal drugs. The question arises whether these phytoconstituents are available commercially or only laboratory level isolation methods are documented. The answer for this question is yes, phytoconstituents are commercially available and few of them are discussed with respect to their industrial method of isolation and utilization in this chapter.

Forskolin

Forskolin is the labdane diterpene extracted from the roots of *Coleus forskohlii* also known as *Plectranthus barbatus* from family- Lamiaceae. It is traditionally used in India for the treatment of high blood pressure, asthma and heart related complications. It is native to India and known as Pashanbhedi as it grows through the rocks. Forskolin is commonly used as a tool in biochemistry to raise levels of cyclic AMP (cAMP) in the study and research of cell physiology. In biogenetic pathway it is derived from geranyleranyl pyrophosphate.

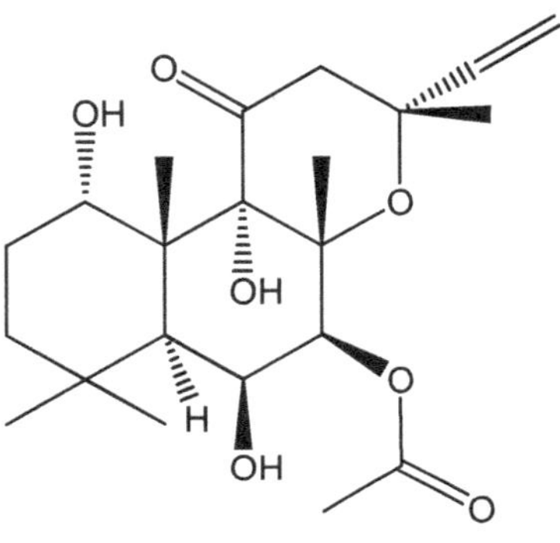

Forskolin

Industrial Production

1. Extract the roots and bark powder of *Coleus forskohlii* with toulene at 60 °C for 2 h with contineous stirring.

2. Filter the solution and concentrate under reduced pressure and temprature below 40 °C

3. Treat the reduced extract with n- hexane which yields brown precipitate of forskolin

4. The crude forskolin is further purified by column chromatography by using silica gel column with solvent mixture of acetonitrile : methanol. The eluted compound is confirmed by TLC.

Estimation of Forskolin

By TLC and HPTLC

Preparation of standard and sample solution: Six gradual increased concentration of standard forskolin prepared in chloroform. Similarly predetermined concentration of isolated forskolin test solution prepared as sample solution.

Stationary phase: Silica Gel GF 254

Mobile phase: Toulene : Ethyl Acetate (8.5:1.5 v/v)

Derivatising agent: Vanilin sulphuric acid reagent

The series of gradual increasing concentraion spots of standard forskolin and known concentration of isolated sample forskolin are applied with TLC applicator on precoated silica gel plate.

TLC plate is developed in presaturated chamber with mobile phase. After ascending development, plate dried and derivatised with vanilin sulphuric acid reagent. For quantitative estimation, derivatised plate is scanned by using densitometer. The calibration curve of peak AUC versus concentrations is plotted and by extrapolating the graph unknown concentration forskolin in sample solution is determined.

Utilization

- Due to vasodilatory and cardiac stimulant effects, it is used in the treatment of hypertension and congestive cardiac failure.
- It reduces intraocular pressure so used in treatment of glaucoma.
- IV infusion used in schizophrenic patients for antidepressant activity.
- It promotes lean body mass and act as anti-obesity agent.

Sennosides

Sennosides are obtained from the dried leaflets of *Cassia acutifolia* (Alexandrain senna) and *Cassia angustifolia* (Indian senna) from family- Leguminosae. Indian senna should contain minimum 2% of sennoside as calcium sennoside.

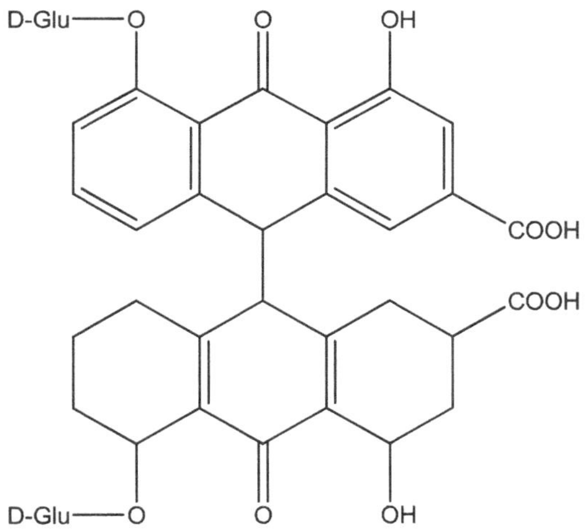

Sennosides

Industrial Production

Method 1

1. Extract 20 gm of powdered senna leaves with benzene for 2 h on an electric shaker.
2. Filter the extract under pressure and distill it to remove traces of solvent.
3. Dry the residue and extract with 70 % methanol (600ml) for 5-6 h.
4. Filter the extract and re-extract with 70 % methanol (400ml) for 2 h.
5. Filter the methanolic extract, pool together and concentrate to $1/8^{th}$ of its volume.
6. Acidify the solution using HCl to pH 3.2 with constant stirring and keep at 5 °C for 2 h.

7. Filter the solution under reduced pressure and to the residue add anhydrous calcium chloride in denatured spirit with continuous stirring.

8. Then basify the solution by adding ammonia solution to maintain pH 8 and keep it aside for 2 h.

9. Sennosides precipitate out, filter the solution and dry the precipitate over diphosphate pentoxide in desiccator.

Method 2

1. Extract the dried senna leaves powder with ethanolic chloroform (chloroform: ethanol; 93:7 v/v) for 1 h.

2. Filter the extract and re extract the marc with acidic methanol (12 g per liter oxalic acid in methanol).

3. Combine both the extracts together, reduce under pressure and keep it aside for 24 h.

4. Sennoside A precipitates out while sennoside B remains in the solution.

5. Filter the precipitated Sennoside A, dry and recrystallize it in trimethylamine.

6. For separation of sennoside B; to the filtrate add 10 % calcium chloride solution.

7. Sennosides precipitates as calcium sennoside. Separate it by using methanolic ammonia solution, wash with water and finally recrystallize with glycol monoethyl ether.

Estimation of Sennosides

BY HPLC

Preparation of standard and test solution

A 0.004% w/v solution of sennoside A & B is considered as reference standard. Sample solution is prepared by extracting 1 g of coarsely powdered senna leaves in round bottom flask with mixture of 10 ml acetic acid and 25 ml methanol followed by reflux condensation for 30 minutes. Allow to cool and make up the volume with methanol

Experimental conditions:

Column: C 18 (25 cm × 4.5 cm)

Column packing: octadecylsilane bonded to porous silica

Mobile phase: 1 % v/v acetic acid in water: acetonitrile (82:18 v/v)

Flow rate: 1 ml/min

Detection: 350 nm

Both the sample solution and standard solution are injected and the content of the sennoside A and B are calculated

Utilization:

- Senna is used in treating constipation, it acts by stimulating intestinal peristalsis.
- It is useful in painful hemorrhoids, as it ensures soft and easy bowel movements.
- It also used in treatment of various skin diseases like acne, eczema.
- It is useful in loss of appetite, dysentery, hepatomegaly, indigestion, gout, rheumatism.

Artemisinin

It is a sesquiterpene lactone obtained from the leaves and closed unexpanded flower heads of *Artemisia annua*; family-Astreaceae. Artemisinin and its semisynthetic derivatives found to be very active against the plasmodium species (*P. falciperum, P. vivax, P. malariae*). Chemically it contains an unusual peroxide bridge, its endoperoxide ring is responsible for the activity.

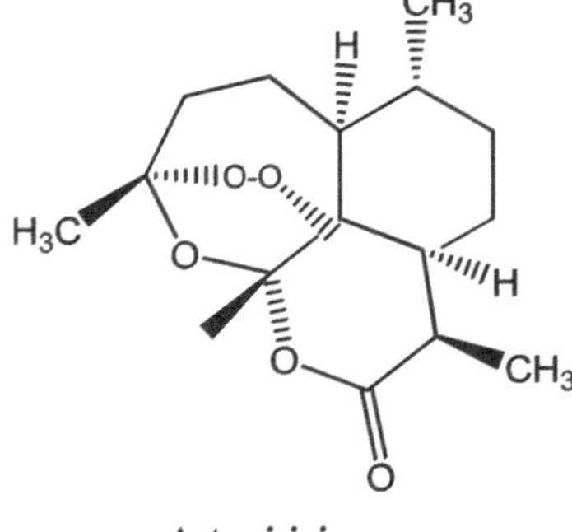

Artemisinin

Industrial Production

1. Powder the dried leaves of *Artemisia annua* and extract with methanol using kinetic maceration technique.
2. Repeat the kinetic maceration many times till the methanol becomes colorless.
3. Pool the methanol extracts together and reduced 100 ml under vacuum at 40 °C and partition this extract with hexane several times till the hexane layer become colorless.
4. Now two fractions are separated; methanolic and hexane fraction.
5. To the methanol fraction add little amount of water to make it hydroalcoholic. Partition this hydroalcoholic extract with ethyl acetate.
6. Repeat the process several times till the ethyl acetate layer is colorless.
7. Separate these two fractions, ethyl acetate fraction is semi polar and hydroalcoholic fraction is polar fraction. Reduce both fractions under vacuum at 40°C separately
8. The most viscous extract (polar) contains artemisinin.
9. Fractionate the extract by column chromatography using gradient elution technique.
10. Collect each separated fraction in column separately and identify for the presence of artemisinin by TLC.
11. The fractions showing presence of artemisinin is then used for preparative TLC to obtain artemisinin.

Estimation / Analysis of Artemisinin

Estimation by HPLC

A series of solutions of known concentrations of artemisinin and predetermined concentration of *A. annua* extract samples are prepared for the analysis of artemisinin in plant extract by reverse phase liquid chromatography. C_{18} column is used as stationary phase while formic acid (% 0.2 v/v): acetonitrile (50:50v/v) is used as mobile phase. The isocratic elution technique is chosen to achieve maximum separation and sensitivity by maintaining flow rate 1.0 ml/min. The samples were detected at 254 nm using photodiode array detector. Results of artemisinin quantities in Artemisia samples were expressed as the mean of three determinations by using calibration curve.

Estimation by HPTLC

The known concentration of hexane extract of *A. annua* is used as test solution while standard artemisinin of known purity and known concentration dissolved in hexane is used as standard solution. The TLC plate is developed using mobile phase n-Hexane: Ethyl Acetate (75:25, v/v) in a saturated chamber. After development plate is derivatized with anisaldehyde-sulphuric acid reagent followed by heating at 110°C for 10 min. The presence of pink color spot at *Rf* 0.28 confirms the presence of artemisinin. Similarly, the plate is scanned using HPTLC densitometer at 540 nm. By using calibration curve the quantity of the artemisinin in sample is calculated.

Utilization

- Artemisinin is used as an antimalarial drug which exerts cidal activity towards the blood schizonts of the parasite.

- It is a first line therapy for *P.falciperum* malaria worldwide. As it is having very short half life it is used in Artemisinin combination therapy (ACT) with one or two long acting drugs like amodiaquin/mefloquine.

- Artemisinin derivative artesunate is considered superior to quinine in treatment of malaria through parental administration.

- Artemisinin and its derivatives are known to suppress the inflammatory immune reactions.

Diosgenin

Diosgenin commercially obtained from the tubers of *Dioscorea deltoida, D. compositae*; family-Dioscoriaceae. It is commonly known as Yam-used as vegetable.

Chemically it is aglycone portion i.e. phytosteroid sapogenin obtained after the hydrolysis of steroidal saponin glycoside dioscin present in dioscoria. Glycosides are soluble in polar solvents while the aglycone portion obtained after hydrolysis is soluble in nonpolar solvents. These solubility parameters are the basic behind isolation of glycoside.

Diosgenin

Industrial Production

By Acid Hydrolysis

1. Powder the Dioscorea tubers coarsely and dry in sun.
2. Mix The tuber powder with 2.5 N sulphuric acid and reflux for 1 h.
3. The hydrolysis of glycosides takes place. Filter this hydrolyzed mixture.
4. Concentrate the filtrate and extract with non- polar solvent viz. benzene.
5. Reduce the benzene extract under pressure and recrystallize diosgenin by acetone.

By Alcoholic Extraction Followed by Acid Hydrolysis

1. Powder the Dioscorea tubers coarsely and dry it in sun.
2. Extract the tuber powder with ethanol or methanol for 6-8 h. Later collect the alcohol extract and reduce to syrupy consistency.
3. Hydrolyze the syrupy extract by using sulphuric acid for 6-12 h.
4. The hydrolysis results into conversion of dioscin into diosgenin which precipitate out.
5. Filter The precipitate wash and purify with alcohol.

By Fermentation Followed by Acid Hydrolysis

1. Powder the fresh tubers and keep in fermentation bin for fermentation for 2 days.
2. Dry the fermented material under sun till the moisture content is less than 8 %.
3. The dried tuber powder is then subject to reflux condensation with sulphuric acid for 4-5 h.
4. Neutralize the resulting marc by addition of alkali and wash several times with water.
5. Dry the neutralized marc and extract with heptanes to isolate diosgenin.

Estimation of Diosgenin

By HPTLC

Preparation of standard and sample solution: Six gradually increasing concentrations of standard diosgenin are prepared in methanol. Similarly predetermined concentration of isolated diosgenin solution is prepared and used as a sample solution.

Stationary phase: Silica gel F 254

Mobile phase: n- Hexane: Ethyl acetate (4:2 v/v)

Derivatizing agent: 3g of antimony chloride in 100 ml hydrochloric acid.

The different concentration of standard solution and sample solution is applied on precoated silica gel F 254 HPTLC plates and allow to develop in pre-saturated TLC chamber. After ascending development, plates are dried and derivatized. Diosgenin shows green black color spot. For quantitative estimation derivatized plates are scanned using densitometer. The calibration curve of peak AUC versus standard diosgenin concentrations is plotted and then AUC of test sample extrapolated on calibration curve to quantify it.

Utilization

- Diosgenin is used as a precursor for the synthesis of various corticosteroids, oral contraceptives and sex hormones.
- Diosgenin is used in the treatment of rheumatoid arthritis.
- Used in hormone replacement therapy.
- Diosgenin may behave as prodrug to progesterone.

Digoxin

Digoxin is obtained from the dried leaves of *Digitalis lanata* or *Digitalis purpurea* (famiy-Scrophulariaceae). Digoxin is a secondary glycoside produced from primary glycoside lanatoside C. *Digitalis lanata* contains more amount of digoxin. *D. lanata* contains primary glycosides Lanatoside A, B and C. On mild hydrolysis lanatoside C seperates the glucose leaving behind secondary glycoside digoxin.

Digoxin

Digitoxin

Industrial production

Method 1

1. Powder the leaves of *D. lanata* and extract with 50% methanol at low temperature.
2. Filter the extract and add lead acetate to the filtrate for the removal of impurities.
3. Centrifuge the solution and decant the supernatant liquid.
4. Extract the supernatant with chloroform, evaporate the chloroform extract.
5. Purify the residue left behind by chromatography for the digoxin.

Method 2

1. The fresh leaves of *D. lanata* convert into paste form and treat with neutral salts to inactivate oxidase enzyme which converts glycoside to aglycone portion.

2. Defat the salt treated portion with benzene and extract with ethyl acetate.

3. The resultant extract contains the lanatoside C which can be further purified by chromatography.

4. The purified lanatoside C on hydrolysis yields digoxin.

Estimation of Digoxin

By UV spectrophotometry (IP method)

Preparation of test and standard solution: weigh accurately about 40 mg of test and standard digoxin in sufficient ethanol (95 %) to produce 50 ml. Dilute the 5 ml solution from stock solution to 100 ml with the same solvent.

Assay

- To 5 ml of the resulting solution add 3 ml of alkaline picric acid solution. Allow to stand for 30 min. in subdued light.

- Measure the absorbance of the solution at 495 nm.

- Perform blank measurements without sample/ test solution.

- Calculate the content of the digoxin from the absorbance of standard and test solutions.

- % Assay = (sample abs./standard abs.) × (standard conc./sample conc.)

Utilization of Digoxin

- Digoxin is used as a cardiotonic.

- Digoxin is used to treat heart failure.

- Also used to treat atrial fibrillation.

Atropine

Atropine is a tropane alkaloid obtained from dried leaves of *Atropa belladonna* (European belladonna) or *Atropa accuminata* (Indian belladona); family- Solanaceae. It is commonly known as belladonna or deadly night shade leaf.

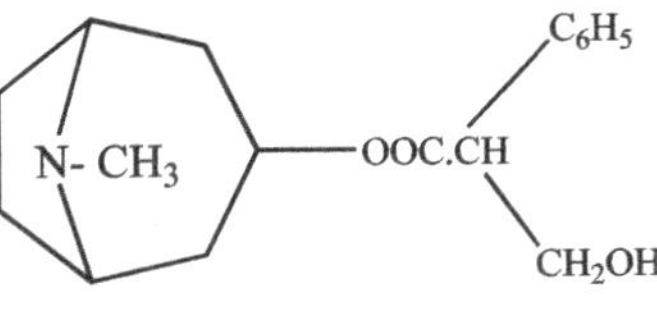

Atropine

Atropine is very soluble in ethanol, slightly soluble in chloroform.

Industrial Production

Method 1

1. First extract the drug material in powdered form with ethanol.

2. Filter and evaporate the solvent to yield syrupy extract. Treat the extract with dilute hydrochloric acid in order to form alkaloidal salt, and resinous matter will get precipitate out

3. Filter the solution; resinous matter retained on the filter paper.

4. Partition the acidic solution with petroleum ether/ chloroform in a separating funnel.

5. Collect the chloroform/ petroleum ether layer and remove by distillation to get the crude alkaloidal mixture which is further treated with oxalic acid.

6. Separate the oxalates of atropine and hyoscyamine by fractional crystallization from acetone and ether which gives the atropine oxalates crystals.

Method 2

1. Extract the aerial parts and roots of belladonna with ethanol.

2. Heat the obtained extract with potassium carbonate solution which converts hyoscyamine to atropine

3. Partition the alkaline extract with organic solvent like chloroform.

4. Concentrate the chloroform extract and further partition it with dilute sulphuric acid to get acidic fraction.

5. Make the acidic fraction alkaline with potassium carbonate which results into the precipitation of atropine.

6. Filtered the precipitate, wash and dissolve in ether and convert to oxalate or sulphate by treating with respective acids.

Estimation of Atropine

Assay of atropine sulphate by titrimetric method

The atropine content as atropine sulphate is determined by titrimetric method. The accurately weighed quantity of test solution i.e. sulphate salt dissolved in 50 ml of glacial acetic acid and titrated with 0.1 N perchloric acid and endpoint is determined by potentiometry.

The blank determination is also carried out and the amount of atropine sulphate is calculated by using the factor;

Each ml of 0.1 N perchloric acid is equivalent to 0.06770 g of atropine sulphate.

By TLC

Standard solution: 1% solution of atropine is added to 2 N acetic acid

Stationary phase: Silica gel G

Mobile phase: Strong ammonia solution: methanol (1.5: 100)

Derivatizing agent: Dragendorffs reagent

Rf value: 0.18

Utilization

- Atropine is used as a mydriatic to dilate pupil of the eye.

- Also use to reduce the secretions like saliva, tears, sweat, and gastric juices.

- It is used as antidote in pilocarpine poisoning.

- It is also administered intravenously for the treatment of bradycardia.

- It is used as pre-anesthetic medication.

Podophyllotoxin

Podophyllotoxin is a lignin derivative of podophyllin a resinous matter obtained from dried roots and rhizomes of *Podophyllum peltatum* (American podophyllum) and *Podophyllum hexandrum* (Indian podophyllum); family-Berberidaceae. The resin should contain not less than 40 % of podophyllotoxin.

Podophyllotoxin is insoluble in ethyl ether, slightly soluble in water, soluble in acetone, benzene and very soluble in ethanol and chloroform.

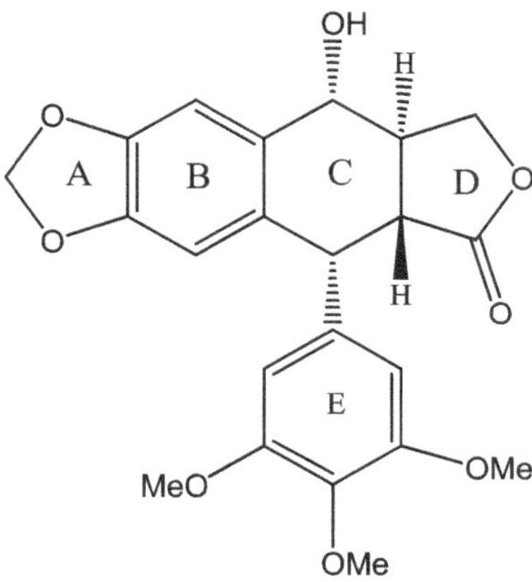

Podophyllotoxin

Industrial Production of Podophyllotoxin

1. Extract the powdered podophyllum with methanol in Soxhlet extractor.
2. Filter the extract and reduce the volume under reduced pressure to syrupy consistency.
3. To this add very dilute hydrochloric acid (10 ml diluted to 100 ml) and keep aside for 30 minutes.
4. Resinous matter precipitates, filter the solution and wash the resin several times with cold water.
5. After drying brown colored precipitate of podophyllin can be obtained.
6. Dissolve the residue in sufficient quantity of hot 90% ethanol, filter and evaporate to dryness.
7. Recrystallize the residue in benzene to yield podophyllotoxin.

Estimation of Podophyllotoxin

By TLC

Stationary phase: Silica gel G coated TLC plate

Mobile phase: Toulene:Ethyl acetate (5:7 v/v)

Sample and standard solution preparation: 1mg /ml solution of both standard podophyllotoxin and podophyllum extract is prepared in methanol.

The standard and sample solutions are spotted on TLC plates and kept in already saturated chamber for development. After development plate is dried and sprayed with sulphuric acid solution.

Rf value for podophyllotoxin is 0.39

Utilization of podophyllotoxin

- Podophyllin shows cytotoxic activity hence it is used for the treatment of venereal and other warts.

- Podophyllotoxin is used as a precursor for semisynthetic anticancer drugs like etoposide and teniposide which is mainly used for the treatment of lung, ovarian and testicular cancer.

- Podophyllum resin is a strong gastrointestinal irritant and acts as a drastic purgative

- Podophyllotoxin cream is commonly prescribed as a potent topical antiviral for the treatment of HPV infections with external warts.

Caffeine

Caffeine is a methylated xanthene alkaloid derivative obtained from the tea plant (*Thea sinensis*; family- Theaceae) and coffee beans (*caffea arabica*; family- Rubiaceae). The caffeine percentage in coffee beans found around 1-2 % while in tea leave 1-5 %.

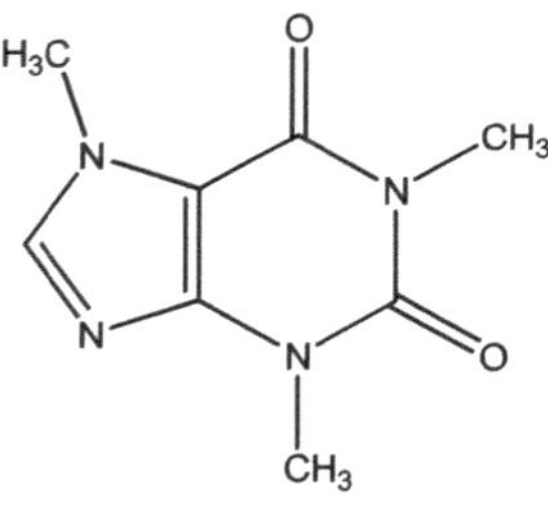

Caffeine

Caffeine can be isolated from cocoa seeds (*Theobroma cacao*; family-Sterculiaceae), Kola seeds (*cola acuminate*; family-Sterculiaceae).In general isolation of caffeine is done by using tea leaves powder. Other than alkaloids tea leaves contain cellulose, tannins and chlorophyll. Caffeine is highly soluble in dichloromethane and also soluble in hot water.

Industrial Production of Caffeine

1. Take about 30 g of tea leaves; to this add 250 ml of water. Also add 5 g of sodium carbonate in the solution to remove the tannins.

2. Boil the solution for 10 min.

3. Filter the solution while hot

4. Extract the marc with 100 ml of water

5. Combine the water extracts and allow to cool.

6. Partition the water extract with 25 ml of dichloromethane in a separating funnel.

7. Collect the dichloromethane layer

8. Repeat the process again 2 times to ensure complete extraction and combine the extracts.

9. Filter the dichloromethane extract through the bed of anhydrous sodium carbonate packed on glass funnel with cotton wool to remove any moisture present.

10. Evaporate dichloromethane, silky crystals of caffeine are observed which can be recrystallized by using hot ethanol.

Estimation of Caffeine

By Titrimetric Assay method (IP)

Weigh accurately isolated purified caffeine as specified and dissolve it in 5 ml of anhydrous glacial acetic acid with gentle heat. The mixture is titrated with 0.1 m perchloric acid and determine the end point by potentiometry. The percentage content calculated by using factor; 1 ml of 0.1M perchloric acid is equivalent to 0.01942 g of caffeine.

By TLC

Stationary phase: Silica gel G coated TLC plate

Mobile phase: Ethyl acetate: methanol: acetic acid (80:10:10 v/v/v)

Sample and standard solution preparation: 1mg /ml solution of both standard caffeine and tea leaves extract is prepared in methanol.

The standard and sample solutions are spotted on TLC plates and kept in already saturated chamber for development. After development plate is dried and sprayed with Dragendroffs reagent.

Rf value for caffeine is 0.41

Utilization of Caffeine

- Caffeine acts as a CNS stimulant, mild diuretic and prescribed for the treatment of migraine with ergotamine and with aspirin for analgesic effect.

Taxol

Taxol is a diterpenoid pseudo alkaloid obtained from the bark of *Taxus brevifolia;* family-Taxaceae. Taxol is hydrophobic in nature.

Taxol

Industrial production of Taxol

Method 1

1. Extract the powdered bark of *Taxus* plant with methanol exhaustively.
2. Filter the extract and evaporate to dryness at temperature below 40 °C. Discard the marc.
3. The dried extract partition with the mixture of carbon tetrachloride and water several times.
4. Collect the carbon tetrachloride fractions and evaporate to dryness at temperature below 40°C.
5. Again, extract the dried carbon tetrachloride fraction residue with mixture of carbon tetrachloride: methanol (1:1).
6. Filter the fraction and evaporate to dryness to obtain crude taxol.
7. The crude taxol can be further purified by TLC.

Method 2: Plant tissue culture

1. Callus culture is prepared from yew plant cells of young stem on the Gamborge's B-5 agar medium.
2. By using plant tissue culture considerable amount of taxol can be produced.
3. The individual separated plant cells from the callus suspended in liquid broth in different bioreactor and taxol can be produced as static suspension culture or continuous suspension culture.
4. In the continuous culture, the outflow of the liquid broth is maintained with inflow of fresh broth and thus continuous production of taxol can be achieved.

Estimation of Taxol

By HPLC

Preparation of standard and sample solution: known concentrations of test and standard Taxol solutions are prepared in methanol.

Stationary phase: 30cm×3.9mm column, packed in pentafluro phenyl group chemically bonded to porous silica.

Mobile phase: Water: acetonitrile (11:9)

Flow rate: 1.5ml/min

Detection wavelength: 227 nm

By comparing the AUC of test and standard calculate the content of taxol in sample

BY HPTLC

Stationary phase: Chloroform: Methanol (7:1v/v)

Mobile phase: Silica gel F254

Visualizing agent: vanillin sulphuric acid reagent

The series of gradually increasing concentrations of standard taxol spotted on precoated silica gel plates along with known concentration of sample of taxol. After ascending development in presaturated TLC chamber the plate is derivatized with vanillin sulphuric acid reagent and heated at 110 °C for 10 minutes. Blue spots appear. The calibration curve of AUC versus concentration of standard taxol used to quantify the taxol in test solution.

Utilization

- Taxol is an approved drug for the treatment of ovarian, breast, lung, bladder, prostate, melanoma, esophageal and other types of solid tumor cancers.

- It is also used as an antiproliferative agent for the prevention of restenosis of coronary and peripheral stents.

Vincristine And Vinblastine

Vincristine and Vinblastine are indole alkaloids obtained from the aerial parts of the plant *Catharanthus roseus*; family-Apocynaceae, commonly known as periwinkle or vinca. The percentage of these alkaloids in vinca is very less around 0.04 %. These are highly potent antineoplastic phytoconstituents.

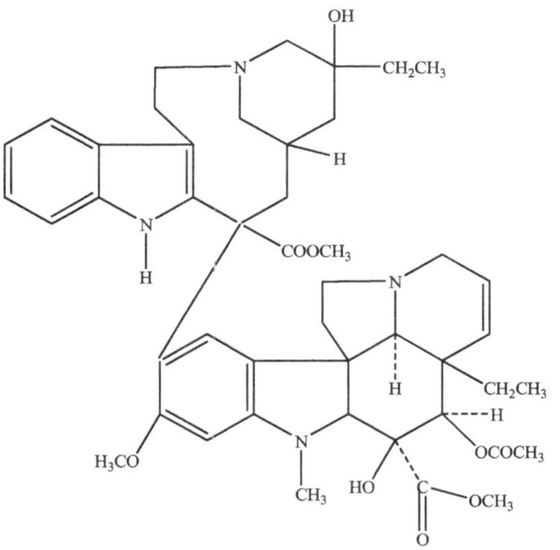

Vinblastin

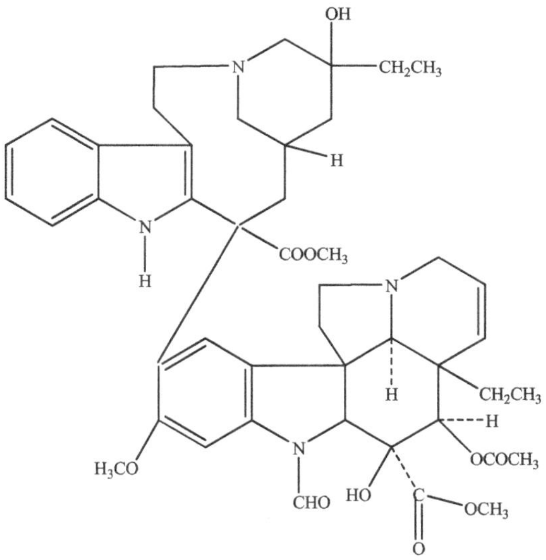

Vincristine

Industrial Production of Vincristine and Vinblastine

Method 1

1. Extract the dried vinca leaves with aqueous alcoholic acetic acid solution (1:9:1 v/v).

2. Concentrate the aqueous extract and the residue further extract with 2% hydrochloric acid.

3. Adjust the pH of this acid extract 4 by sodium hydroxide solution and then extract with benzene.

4. Again, raise the pH to 7 and again extract with benzene to separate alkaloids.

5. Mix the benzene extracts together, concentrate, dry and dissolve in benzene: methylene chloride (65:35 v/v) solvent.

6. Further can be subjected to chromatographic separation to separate vincristine and vinblastine.

Method 2

- Vincristine and vinblastine can be produced by plant tissue culture technique.

- Young leaves and flowering shoots of vinca plant are used as a source of callus culture. The subculturing is done after 4 weeks of initiation followed by subsequent subculturing after every 3 weeks.

- To increase the alkaloid concentration, the Zenk medium is used and it is prepared by using 50 % glucose, 2.5 % gelrite, 1 µM kinetin and other essential nutrients. The media is sterilized and the experiment is carried out in aseptic area with sterilized equipment.

- Callus collected on day 8 and 11 are freeze dried, powdered and extracted with methanol.

- This methanol extract is then used for isolation of vincristine and vinblastine.

Estimation of Vincristine and Vinblastine

By TLC

Stationary phase: Silica gel G coated TLC plate.

Mobile phase: Acetonitrile: benzene (30:70 v/v).

Sample and standard solution preparation: 1mg /ml solution of both standard vincristine and vinblastine extract is prepared in methanol.

The standard and sample solutions are spotted on TLC plates and kept in already saturated chamber for ascending development. After development plate is dried and sprayed with1 % cerric ammonium sulphate solution in 85 % phosphoric acid. The *Rf* value of vincristine is 0.39.

Utilization of Vincristine and Vinblastine

- Vinblastine is an antitumour alkaloid used in the treatment of Hodgkin's disease

- Vincristine is used in treatment of non-Hodgkin's lymphoma, Hodgkin's lymphoma, acute lymphoblastic leukemia.

- Vincristine and Vinblastine are used intravenously for various types of chemotherapy regimens. It is also used in the treatment of diabetes.

Probable Questions

Long answer questions

1. Write the method of industrial isolation and commercial utilization of sennosides.

2. Explain the method of industrial isolation, estimation and commercial utilization of important cardiac glycoside.

3. Write the steps involved in commercial method of isolation of forskolin.

Short answer questions

1. Write the industrial isolation method of any one of the alkaloid.
2. Explain the estimation method of taxol.
3. Explain industrial isolation of vincristine.
4. Write a short note isolation of diosgenin.

Very short answer questions

1. Write structure of diosgenin and digoxin.
2. Write the commercial utilization of taxol.
3. Explain the commercial use of vinca alkaloids.
4. Write anyone estimation method of artemisinin.
5. Write the structure and commercial use of podophyllotoxin.

Unit V

Basics of Phytochemistry

PCI Syllabus

Basics of Phytochemistry; Modern methods of extraction, application of latest techniques like Spectroscopy, chromatography and electrophoresis in the isolation, purification and identification of crude drugs.

Book Chapter Contents

Pphytochemistry

- Introduction to Extraction
  - Conventional methods of Extraction.
- Recent / Modern Methods of Extraction
  - Continuous hot extraction (Soxhlet Extraction)
  - Supercritical Fluid Extraction
  - Microwave assisted Extraction
- Analytical Techniques Used in Isolation, Purification and Identification of crude drugs
- Chromatography Introduction
  - Thin Layer Chromatography (TLC)
  - High Performance Thin Layer Chromatography (HPTLC)
  - Column Chromatography
  - High performance Liquid chromatography (HPLC)
  - Gas Chromatography
- Spectroscopy introduction
  - UV/Visible Spectroscopy
  - Infra-Red Spectroscopy
  - Mass Spectroscopy
  - Nuclear Magnetic Resonance Spectroscopy
  - Electrophoresis

Phytochemistry

Phytochemistry is the study of phytochemicals means chemical constituents derived from plants. Phytochemistry helps to describe the chemistry of the large number of primary and secondary metabolites found in plants, the functions of these compounds in human and plant biology, and the biosynthesis of these compounds in plants. Plants synthesize phytochemicals for many reasons, including protecting themselves against insect's attack and certain plant diseases. Phytochemicals in food plants are often plays an active role in human biology and in many cases have health benefits. The compounds found in plants are chemically different but most common chemical forms found are the alkaloids, glycosides, polyphenols, and terpenes. These chemical compounds have enormous effects on human health. Research has shown that the individual chemical entity isolated from plants gives better results than synthetically derived drugs. As a result of this the demand for isolated compounds has increased. New methods, techniques are being developed by the research scientists daily. Techniques commonly used in the field of phytochemistry are extraction, isolation, chromatography and different types of spectroscopy.

Extraction

Extraction is a process in which the physical separation of phytoconstituents takes place which are in the insoluble plant matrix. This process of solubilization takes place with help of water or with the help of polar to nonpolar organic solvents. This solvent is known as **menstrum** whereas the solution containing the extracted phytoconstituents is known as **miscella** and the insoluble material after exhausting / extraction the drug is known as **marc**.

In brief extraction can be defined as "the process in which the animal or plant tissues are treated with specific solvents whereby the medicinally active constituents are dissolved out, cell tissues and most of inert components remain undissolved"

Mechanism of Extraction

Solid extraction by using appropriate solvent, is most preferred method for extraction of phytoconstituent from plant material. In this method, firstly solvent penetrates into the solid matrix, then the solubilization of solute in solvent takes place. Later the solute diffuses out of the solid matrix and finally extracted solutes are separated out by solvent evaporation method.

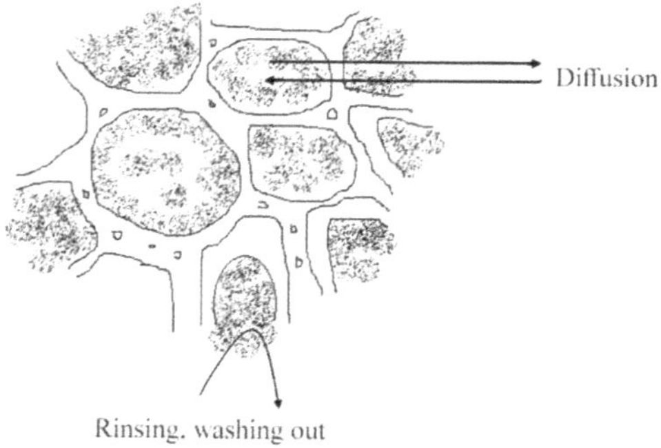

Fig. 5.1 Mechanism of extraction

Factors affecting extraction efficiency

1. **Menstrum:** The extraction process based upon the principle like dissolves like. Hence polar solvents are appropriate for the extraction of polar secondary metabolite and nonpolar solvents are useful for extraction of nonpolar secondary metabolite.

2. **Plant particle size:** Reduced particle size will increase the surface area for the extraction at the same time it will expose cell constituents to extracting solvents. Small particle size enhances solvent penetration and solute diffusion and ultimately results in better extraction.

3. **Menstrum to plant material ratio:** The constant quantity of solvent decreases the extraction rate. The extraction rate decreases as solvent get saturated with the phytoconstituents. This can be solved by introducing fixed amount of solvent after particular time interval.

4. **Temperature:** Increase in temperature, increases the solubility and diffusion of phytoconstituents. The temperature at which extraction process is carried out should be observed very critically. Excessive increase in the temperature will result in loss of solvent and may have detrimental effect on phytoconstituents. This should be particularly observed in case of thermo labile phytoconstituents and volatile oils.

5. **Duration of extraction:** Increase in duration of extraction in a certain time range can surely improve the extraction efficiency. Once complete extraction of phytoconstituents is completed increase in the duration of extraction will not have any effect on extraction efficiency.

Ideal properties of the solvents used for extraction

- It should be highly selective for the compound to be extracted.
- It should not react with the extracted compound or with other compounds in the plant material
- It should be economical.
- It should be harmless to human and to the environment.
- It should be completely volatile.
- It should not mix up with water.
- The density of solvent should be different from water density.
- It should have the minimum viscosity.

Conventional or Traditional Methods of Extraction

1. **Infusion**: Fresh infusions are prepared by macerating the crude drug for a short period of time with cold or boiling water. This process consists of treating vegetable crude drugs with boiling water but the drugs are not boiled with the menstrum. These are dilute solutions of the readily soluble constituents of crude drugs.

   Types of Infusion

   Concentrated Infusion: Example- concentrated infusion of Quassia.

   Fresh Infusion: Example- infusion of orange.

2. **Decoction:** In this process, the crude drug is boiled in a specified volume of water for a defined time; it is then cooled and strained or filtered. This procedure is suitable for extracting water-soluble, heat stable constituents. Example -Tea, Coffee decoction differs from infusion in the way that the crude drugs in infusion are not boiled with the menstrum but only boiling menstrum is poured on the drug.

3. **Digestion:** This is a form of maceration in which gentle heat is used during the process of extraction. It is used when moderately elevated temperature is not objectionable. The solvent efficiency of the menstrum is thereby increased. e.g. Extraction of Morphine.

4. **Maceration:** In this process solid ingredients are placed in a stoppered container with the whole solvent and allowed to stand for a period of at least 3 days (3 - 7 days) with frequent agitation, until soluble matter is dissolved. The mixture is then strained (through sieves / nets), the marc pressed and the combined liquids clarified (cleaned byfiltration) or by decantation, after standing. This is the official method mentioned in pharmacopoeias.

   This process is generally used for the preparation of tinctures or extracts and menestrum is usually alcoholic, hydroalcoholic or may be aqueous. This process is carried out at ambient temperature.

   Simple maceration: The extraction of the drug takes place with a solvent with several daily shakings or stirrings at room temperature. In this type of maceration, organized drugs are used. Simple maceration can be categorized as;

   Kinetic maceration: It is carried out at room temperature, like simple maceration, the difference being that the material is kept in constant motion. Generally electronic shakers are used.

   Double/ Triple maceration: Repeated maceration is more effective than a single maceration. The type of drug to be extracted i.e. organized or unorganized decides the need of double/ triple/ multiple maceration. After simple maceration considerable amount of phyto constituents remains in the marc; then drug is again subjected to double or triple maceration. Sometimes when the crude drugs cannot be pressed then triple or multiple maceration is adopted.

5. **Percolation:** Percolation is also an official method of extraction. A percolator which is a narrow, cone-shaped vessel open at both ends is generally used. It is the method of short successive maceration or process of displacement. Generally used to extract active ingredients in the preparation of tinctures and fluid extracts. It is continuous downward displacement of the solvent through the bed of crude drug material to get extract.

Steps involved in percolation:

Size reduction: The drug to be extracted is subjected to suitable degree of size reduction, usually from coarse powder to fine powder.

Imbibition: Imbibition is the process in which the powdered drug is moistened with a suitable amount of menstrum and allowed to stand for four hours in a well closed container.

Packing: After imbibition the moistened drug is evenly packed into the percolator.

Maceration: After packing the crude drug, sufficient menstrum is added to saturate the material.

Percolation: The lower tap is opened and liquid collected therein is allowed to drip slowly at a controlled rate until 3/4th volume of the finished product is obtained.

Percolator: The percolator is a conical vessel with a top opening in which is placed a circular drilled lid allowing the passage of liquid and subjecting the materials placed on it to a slight pressure. The bottom has an adjustable closure to allow passage of the fluid at a convenient rate.

The plant material is moistened prior to their placement in the percolator with a proper amount of menstrum, it is placed in a sealed container and kept aside for approximately four hours.

After that the plant material must be conveniently placed in the percolator so as to allow the even passage of fluid and the complete contact with the plant material. The percolator must be filled with liquid and covered up. The bottom outlet is opened until get a regular dripping and then closes. More menstrum is added to cover all the material and must stand to soak in the percolator closed for 24 h.

After 24 h leave it to drip slowly and add enough menstruum to a proportional volume of 3/4 of the total volume required for the final product. The wet mass is pressed to extract the maximum residual fluid retained and supplemented with sufficient menstrum to get the sufficient volume, it is filtered or clarified by decantation.

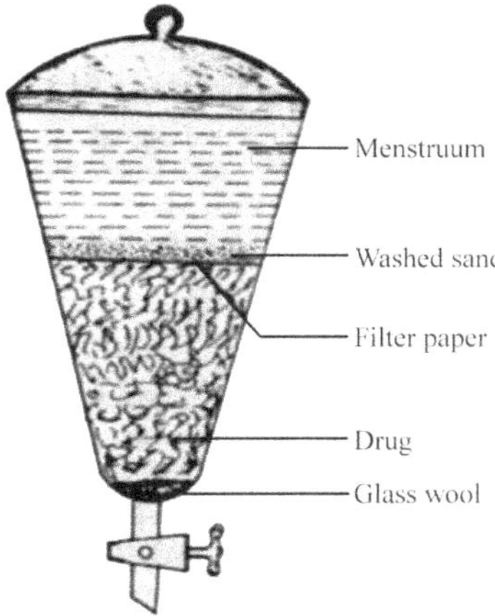

Fig. 5.2 Percolator

Recent / Modern Methods of Extraction
Continuous Hot Percolation / Soxhlet Extraction

When active constituents of the drug are not freely soluble in the solvent or difficult to be displaced from the cells of the drug, then it becomes necessary to extract the crude drug by action of hot menstrum for a considerable length of time. The fixed oils from seeds and alkaloids from the drug are extracted by continuous hot percolation process using benzene, chloroform, petroleum, ether etc.

Soxhlet apparatus: It consist of the following parts,

- Round bottom flask containing the boiling solvent
- Soxhlet Extractor/ thimble: In this the drug to be extracted is packed. It has a side tube which carries the vapors of the solvent from the flask to the condenser and a siphon tube which siphons over the extract from soxhlet extractor to the flask.
- A condenser in which the vapors of the solvent are condensed again into solvent.

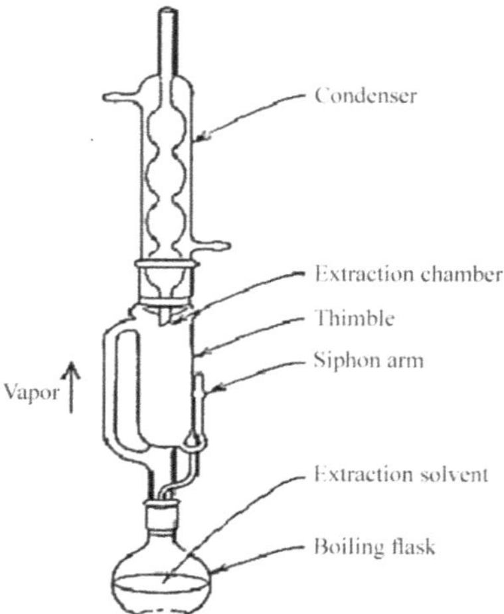

Fig. 5.3 Soxhlet Apparatus

Principle: Soxhlet apparatus performs the extraction by using solvent reflux and siphon principle to continuously extract the solid matrix in presence of pure solvent. It is a continuous hot extraction process which yields high extraction efficiency with minimum use of solvent.

Working: The drug is placed in a thimble packed in a paper cylinder of filter paper. The condenser is fitted with water inlet and outlet. The water tap is opened and tap water is allowed to circulate through condenser. The solvent is placed in the round bottom flask. The apparatus assembly is then fitted as shown in Fig. 5.3. The assembly is then set on heating mantle and switched on the mantle. After reaching the boiling point solvent starts converting into vapors. These vapors enter into the condenser through the side tube and get condensed into hot liquid which falls on the drug placed in thimble. The hot solvents falling on the crude drug starts extracting the active constituents. After certain period the thimble gets filled with the solvent, the excess solvent in the thimble is then siphoned through siphon tube back to the flask. Thus, thimble gets empty and again filled with the solvent coming from condenser. The soluble active constituent of the drug remains in the flask where solvent is repeatedly volatilized. The continuous process of filling and emptying the thimble goes on until the drug is completely exhausted so the method is called as continuous hot extraction method.

Advantages of Soxhlet extractor

- The process is continuous and automatic.
- Soxhlet requires less amount of solvent as it uses the same solvent continuously.
- Less time is required for extraction as compared to other methods.

Disadvantages of Soxhlet extractor:

- This method is not suitable for thermolabile substances as contineous boiling may cause structural changes in them.

- Mixture of two or more solvents cannot be used for extraction as they may have different boiling points.

- The phytoconstituents which are readily soluble in solvent may form precipitate on continuous boiling and hence requires more amount of solvent to dissolve that precipitate afterwards.

Supercritical Fluid Extraction (SFE)

Supercritical fluid extraction (SFE) is method of extraction in which separation of component takes place from the matrix by using supercritical fluid as extracting solvent.

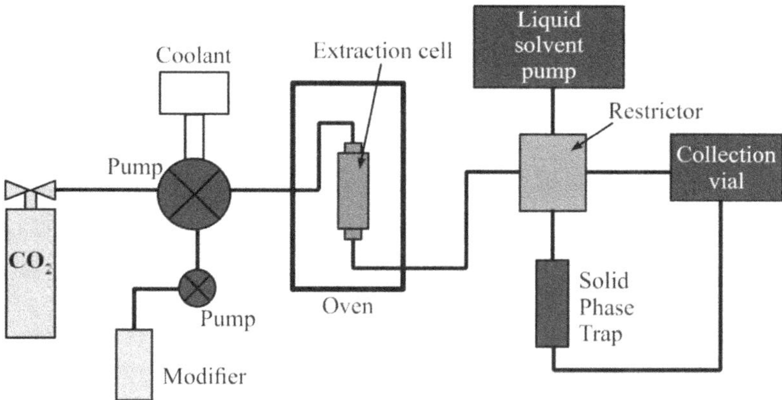

Fig. 5.4 Supercritical fluid extraction (SFE)

A supercritical fluid is any substance at a temperature and pressure above its critical point (the end point of a phase equilibrium curve / above its critical temperature and critical pressure), where distinctive liquid and gas phases do not exist. It can diffuse through solid like a gas, but dissolve phytoconstituents like liquid hence extraction rate can be enhanced. It also reduces the thermal degradation of the important phytoconstituents.

Slight manipulation in pressure or temperature near to critical point of the solvent results in large changes in density hence good solvent power at high densities to very low solvent power at low densities can be achieved.

Supercritical carbon dioxide is the most widely used supercritical fluid for extraction purpose. Extraction conditions for super critical carbon dioxide are above the critical temperature of 31°C and critical pressure of 74 bar. Supercritical fluid is produced by warming gas or liquid on the temperature higher than its critical pressure. Above the critical temperature and pressure, the material exists in one condensed state with properties between gas and liquid. In general term, supercritical fluids have properties between those of a gas and a liquid.

Working of SFE

Schematic diagram of SFE is shown in figure 5.4. The essential components for carrying out supercritical fluid extraction are; a high-pressure extractor, a pressure reduction valve, a low-pressure separator and pump for intensifying the pressure of recycled solvent. The feed i.e. powdered solid material is placed into an extractor. CO_2 is fed to extractor through a high-pressure pump (100 to 350 bar) where the extraction of phytoconstituents take place. From the extractor, CO_2 along with extracted phytoconstituents is sent to a separator (120 to 50 bar) via a pressure reduction valve. Due to reduction in temperature pressure, the extract gets precipitated in the separator, at the same time CO_2 free of any extract is recycled to the extractor.

Advantages of SFE

- Fast and efficient method of extraction of phytoconstituents.
- It has low operating cost.
- Thermally labile material can be extracted.
- No residual solvent in extract.
- Easy and safe to operate.
- Isolation and purification is carried out with great precision.

Microwave Assisted Extraction (MAE)

Microwave assisted extraction is of the efficient method which involves extraction of phytoconstituents from crude drugs. MAE allows organic compounds to be extracted more rapidly. Microwaves are form of non-ionizing electromagnetic radiation with wavelengths ranging from 1 meter to 10 mm with frequencies between 300 MHz (1 meter) and 300 GHz (1 millimeter). The prefix 'micro' in the microwave indicates that microwaves are the waves with shorter wavelengths compared to radio waves. Microwaves are made up of two oscillating perpendicular fields which are electrical field and magnetic field. These microwaves can be used as means of energy carrier or for the production of energy. In case of production of energy, microwave directly act on material which is able to absorb a part of electromagnetic energy and transform it into heat. This conversion of electromagnetic energy into heat energy occurs by two mechanisms; Ionic conduction and dipole rotation. Ionic conduction relates with electromagnetic field and dipole rotation with electric field.

Principle of extraction: Irrespective of any drying method used, plants still do contain some moisture. When this moisture inside the plant material gets heated under the influence of microwave it gets evaporated and creates pressure on the cell wall because of swelling of plant cells. This cause the rupturing of cell wall thus facilitate leaching of phytoconstituents from the cell into surrounding solvent. The effect of microwave energy is strongly dependent on the nature higher temperature attained in MAE which increases dehydration of cellulose and reduces its mechanical strength and this inturn helps solvent to access compounds easily inside the cell of both solvent and the solid matrix i.e. crude plant material. Different polarity solvents can be used from heptane to water or combination of solvents to improve the extraction capacity.

Instrumentation and working

Two types of instruments are commercially available and they use different approaches. The most common procedure involves extraction in a closed vessel under controlled pressure and temperature, while an alternative approach is use of open extracting vessel under atmospheric pressure.

1. **Open system:** In this system, extraction is carried out at atmospheric pressure and is named as focused microwave assisted extraction. In this, the extraction temperature determined by boiling point of solvent at that pressure. To prevent the solvent loss due to evaporation, cooling system is provided at the top of extraction vessel.

2. **Closed system:** This is also known as pressurized microwave assisted extraction which is performed under pressure. In this the pressure can reach below 14 bar. This pressure allows temperature above boiling points of the solvents to be raised enhancing both extraction speed and efficiency.

Microwave oven usually consists of the following components:

Magnetron: For the generation of microwave energy

Wave guide: For the propagation of microwave energy from source to the cavity

Cavity: For placing the extraction vessel (reactor) containing sample to be extracted

Circulator: For reflection of homogenization of radiation

Microwave ovens have two types of action as mentioned below:

1. *Mono-Mode cavity*: The mono-mode cavity generates the frequency that excites only the mode of resonance. In this, the sample is placed in the microwave guide where microwaves are focused.

2. *Multi-mode cavity*: In multi-mode cavity the incident wave is able to affect several modes of resonance. This super imposition of modes causes the homogenization of the microwave field.

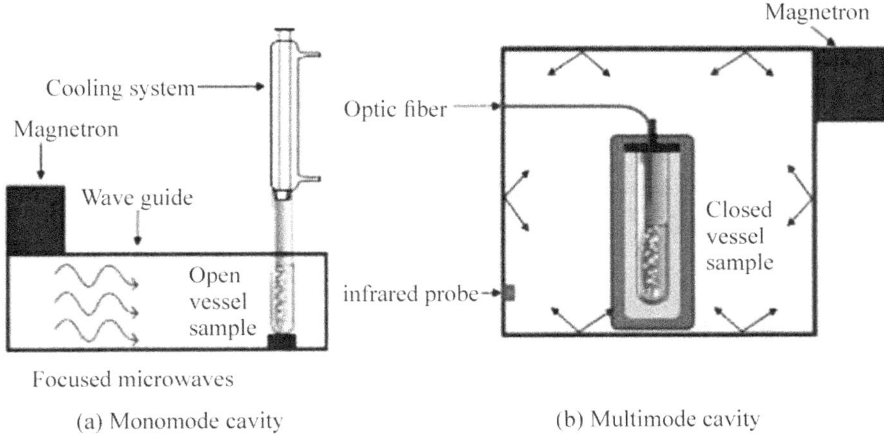

Fig. 5.5 Microwave Oven

Advantages of MAE

- The process is time saving as the extraction process can be completed from few seconds to 15-20 min.

- Less solvent consumption.

- Improve extraction yield.

- The process can be automated precisely hence provide better process accuracy and precision.

- The method is suitable for thermolabile phytoconstituents.

Disadvantages of MAE

- Use of MAE requires specialized setup which increases the cost of process.

- This method is still under the process of development.

Analytical Techniques used in Isolation, Purification and Identification of Crude Drugs

Chromatography

Chromatography is defined as a method of separation of a mixture into individual components through equilibrium distribution between two phases i.e. stationary phase and mobile phase. It is a laboratory technique used for separation of components of a mixture into individual entity. The word 'chromatography' is derived from Greek word *chroma* which means color and graphein which means writing. Chromatography was first employed in Russia in 1900 by the Italian born scientist M. Tswet.

The chromatographic methods involve the following steps:

- Adsorption of substance on stationary phase.

- Separation of adsorbed substance by a mobile phase.

- Recovery of the separated substance by a continuous flow of the mobile phase.

- Qualitative and quantitative analysis of eluted substance.

Types of chromatography

The below mentioned are the types of chromatography:

I. **Based on the nature of stationary and mobile phase**

There are different types of chromatography based on the type of stationary and mobile phase used. They are,

1. **Solid liquid chromatography**: Here stationary phase is solid while mobile phase is liquid. Example- Column chromatography (CC), thin layer chromatography (TLC), high performance liquid chromatography (HPLC).

2. **Liquid liquid chromatography**: Here both stationary and mobile phase used are liquid. Example- paper partition and column partition chromatography.

3. **Gas solid chromatography**: Here stationary phase is gas while mobile phase is solid.

4. **Gas liquid chromatography:** Here stationary phase is gas while mobile phase is liquid.

II. **Based on the principle of separation**

1. **Adsorption chromatography:** When a mixture of compounds dissolved in the mobile phase, it moves through the a column of stationary phase. The compounds travel according to the relative affinities towards the stationary phase. The compound which has more affinity towards stationary phase travels slower and the compound which has lesser affinity towards stationary phase travel faster. Based on the adsorptivity compounds get separated. No two compounds have the same affinity for a combination of stationary and mobile phase. Example- TLC, HPLC.

2. **Partition chromatography:** When two immiscible liquids are present, a mixture of solutes will be distributed according to their partition coefficients. When a mixture of compounds is dissolved in the mobile phase and passed through a column of liquid stationary phase, the component which is more soluble in the stationary phase travels slower. The component which is less soluble in the mobile phase travels faster. Thus, components are separated because of the differences in their partition coefficients. No two components have the same partition coefficients for a particular combination of stationary phase, mobile phase and other conditions.

The stationary phase as such cannot be liquid, hence solid support is used over which a thin film or coating of a liquid is made which acts as a stationary phase.

III. **Based on the modes of chromatography:** Based on the polarity of the stationary phase and mobile phase they are further classified as,

1. **Normal phase chromatography:** In this type stationary phase is polar and mobile phase is non polar.

2. **Reverse phase chromatography:** In this type stationary phase is non polar and mobile phase is polar.

IV. **Other types of chromatography**

1. **Ion Exchange chromatography**: In this type, an ion exchange resin is used. Reversible exchange of ions takes place between similar charged ions and that of ion exchange resin

2. **Gel permeation chromatography**: A gel is used to separate the components of a mixture according to their molecular size. Different gels are used for different molecular weight ranges hence also known as size exclusion chromatography.

3. **Chiral chromatography**: Optical isomers can be separated by using chiral stationary phase.

The important methods of chromatography commonly used in isolation and estimation of phytoconstituents are described in detail below.

Thin Layer Chromatography (TLC)

Principle: TLC is based on the principle of adsorption. When one or more components are spotted on a thin layer of adsorbent coated on a chromatographic plate, the mobile phase solvent flows through because of capillary action. The components move according to their affinities towards the adsorbent i.e. stationary phase. The component with more affinity towards the stationary phase travels slower while the components with lesser affinity towards the stationary phase travels faster. Thus, components get separated on a thin layer of chromatographic plate based on the affinity of the components towards the stationary phase.

Steps involved in TLC: The following steps are involved in TLC

1. **Stationary phase selection:**

    There are several adsorbents which can be used as a stationary phase. Example- Silica gel, Alumina, kieselguhr. As the adsorbent do not adhere to the TLC plate satisfactorily, binder is added to it like gypsum in silica gel G. To visualize the chromatogram after exposure to UV light, fluorescent indicators are added to adsorbent. Example-zinc silicate.

2. **Mobile phase selection:** The mobile phase or solvent system used depends upon various factors-

    *   Nature of component to be separated

    *   Nature of stationary phase used

    *   Mode of chromatography i.e normal or reverse

    *   Separation to be achieved viz. analytical or preparative

    The solvent composition is done by trial and error method along with review of literature and other logical considerations like solubility of substances, polarity of the sample etc.

3. **Chromatographic plate:** Chromatographic plates are glass plates with specific dimensions like 20 x 20 cm (full plate), 20 x 10 cm (half plate) and 20x 5 (quarter plate). These dimensions are used as the width of commercial TLC spreader i.e. 20 cm. Generally during method development microscopic slides are also used. Glass plates of different dimensions can be used if not prepared by using TLC spreader.

4. **Preparation and activation of TLC plates:** The slurry is prepared by mixing adsorbant and water in a particular ratio e.g. Silica gel G and water (1:2). After preparation of slurry the TLC plates are prepared by pouring, dipping, spraying or spreading techniques. TLC spreader is commonly used to prepare uniform thickness of adsorbent on plate. Generally, thickness of plate varies from 0.1 to 0.25 mm. Ready to use or precoated plates are available on glass or plastic sheets. the thickness of these plate is uniform.

    After preparation of TLC plate, activation is done. Activation is nothing but to remove water/ moisture or any adsorbed substances from the surface of the adsorbent. Activation can be achieved by heating at high temperature. Generally, after air drying the plates are heated for 30 minutes in an oven at 110 °C.

5. **Application of sample:** Usually the standard or test sample is spotted on TLC plate by using a capillary tube or micropipette. The spots can be placed at equidistant by using a template with marking. Generally, to get good spot 2-5 μl of the 1 % solution is applied. The spot should be kept at least 2 cm above the base of the plate and spotting area should not be immersed in the mobile phase in development tank.

6. **Preparation of development tank/ TLC chamber**: For the purpose of development a development tank/ chamber is used. It is available in different sizes to hold the TLC plates

of different dimensions. This requires more solvent for developing a chromatogram. When a new method is developed better to use glass beakers to avoid wastage of solvents. In some development tanks at the bottom hump is present because of which solvent required is less. The development tank should be lined inside with the filter paper moistened with mobile phase.

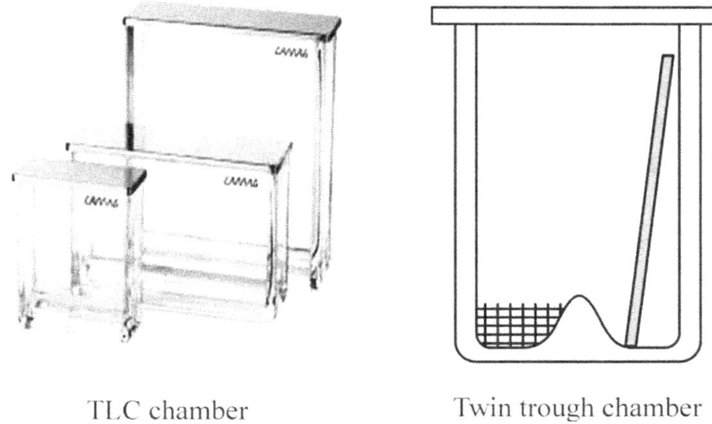

Fig. 5.6 Thin Layer Chromatography

7. **Development techniques:** After spotting different development techniques are used for efficient separation, these are;

- **One dimensional:** In this technique the plates are kept vertical and solvent flows against the gravity because of capillary action

- **Two dimensional:** For complex mixture two dimensional technique is used. First the plates are developed in first axis and after drying developed in the other axis.

- **Multiple development:** In this technique the spotted TLC plate is first developed in one solvent system and after drying again developed in second solvent system. In second solvent system separated spots will further get separated. Generally used in case of closely related compounds.

8. **Detection or visualization:** After the development of TLC plates, the spot should be visualized. The colored spot can be detected visually. But for detecting the colorless spots any one of the following methods can be used.

(a) **Nonspecific methods:** Here the number of spots can be detected but not the exact nature or type of compound.

- **Iodine chamber method:** Here brown or amber spots are observed when TLC plates are kept in a tank few iodine crystals at the bottom.

- **Sulphuric acid spray reagent:** 70-80% v/v of sulphuric acid with few milligrams of potassium dichromate or few mililiter of nitric acid as oxidizing agent is used. This reagent after spraying on TLC plate is heated in oven. Black spots are seen due to charring of compound.

- **UV chamber for fluorescent compound**: When compounds are viewed under UV chamber at 254nm (short) or at 365nm (long) wavelength, fluorescent compound can be detected. Bright spots are seen under dark background.

- **Using fluorescent stationary phase:** When compounds are not fluorescent, a fluorescent stationary phase is used. When the TLC plates are viewed under UV chamber dark spots are seen on fluorescent background.

(b) **Specific methods:** Specific spray reagents or detecting agents are used to find out the nature of compound or for identification like; Ferric chloride for phenolics and tannins, Dragendroff's reagent for alkaloids.

The detecting techniques can also be categorized as,

1. **Destructive technique:** example - specific spray reagent, they destroy the sample after detection

2. **Nondestructive technique:** example - UV chamber, Iodine chamber, here sample is not destroyed even after detection.

9. **Evaluation of chromatogram:** After detecting separated solute, evaluation is done

(a) **Qualitative analysis:** The *Rf* value (Retardation factor) is calculated for identifying the spots i.e. Qualitative analysis.

Rf Value: It is the ratio of distance travelled by solute to the distance travelled by solvent front.

$$Rf = \frac{\text{Distance travelled by solute}}{\text{Distance travelled by solvent front}}$$

Rf value ranges from 0 to 1 but ideal value is in the range of 0.3 to 0.8. The *Rf* value is specific and constant for every compound in particular combination of stationary and mobile phase. When *Rf* value of standard and sample is same, the compound is pure if differs, the compound may different for its reference standard.

(b) **Quantitative analysis:** This can be carried out by using,

Direct method:

- Visual assessment of chromatogram.

- *Determination by measurement of spot areas*: It involves the measurement of shape and size of the spot. It is based upon mathematical relationship between the spot area and amount of substance present. But error may cause because the spot changes during development.

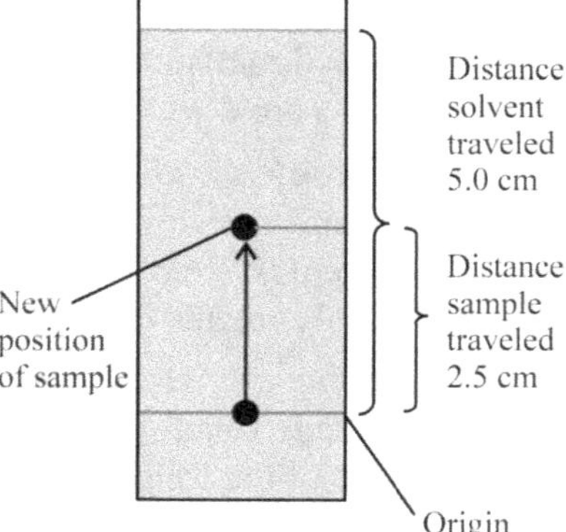

Fig. 5.7 Example of TLC

- *Using densitometer*: Densitometer measures the density of the spots. When the optical density of spots for the standard and sample solutions are measured, the quantity of the substance can be calculated. The plates are neither destroyed nor evaluated with solvents to get compound. This is also known as in situ methods.
- *Direct photometry on TLC*: Characterization of the separated chromatogram zones by reading the absorption or Fluorescence curves directly from TLC plate by using chromatogram spectrophotometer.

Indirect method: It involves the recovery of the separated compound and determination with the suitable instrument. The areas containing the absorbed component are marked and scooped. Then this is dissolved in suitable solvent depending upon the nature of compound. After that adsorbent is separated by centrifugation or filtration. The compound which is present in solvent is then determined by any one of the following techniques like gravimetry, UV spectrophotometry, colorimetry, fluorimetry, etc.

Applications of TLC

- It is used in the isolation and separation of individual components from plant extracts.
- Used for identification of isolated compounds in natural chemistry.
- It helps to determine impurity in the sample.
- Used in the identification of organic compounds.
- It has been used for separating inorganic ions.
- Used for separation of proteins, amino acids.

High Performance Thin Layer Chromatography (HPTLC)

High performance thin layer chromatography is a sophisticated and automated form of TLC. A number of modifications are made to the basic method of TLC to automate the different steps, to increase the resolution and to allow more quantitative measurements. The principle of separation of components in HPTLC is similar to TLC *i.e.* adsorption. The important features of HPTLC are;

- The use of pre coated plates where particle size of stationary phase is uniform and less than 10 μ in diameter.
- Wide choice of stationary phases like silica gel for normal phase and C_{18}, C_8 for reverse phase.
- Auto sampler instead of manual spotting.
- New type of development chambers which requires less amount of solvents for developing.
- More efficient because of smaller and uniform size of adsorbent.
- The use of UV/ visible/fluorescent scanner which scans the entire chromatogram qualitatively and quantitatively.
- The scanner is advanced type of densitometer.
- Improved data processing capabilities by the use of computers.

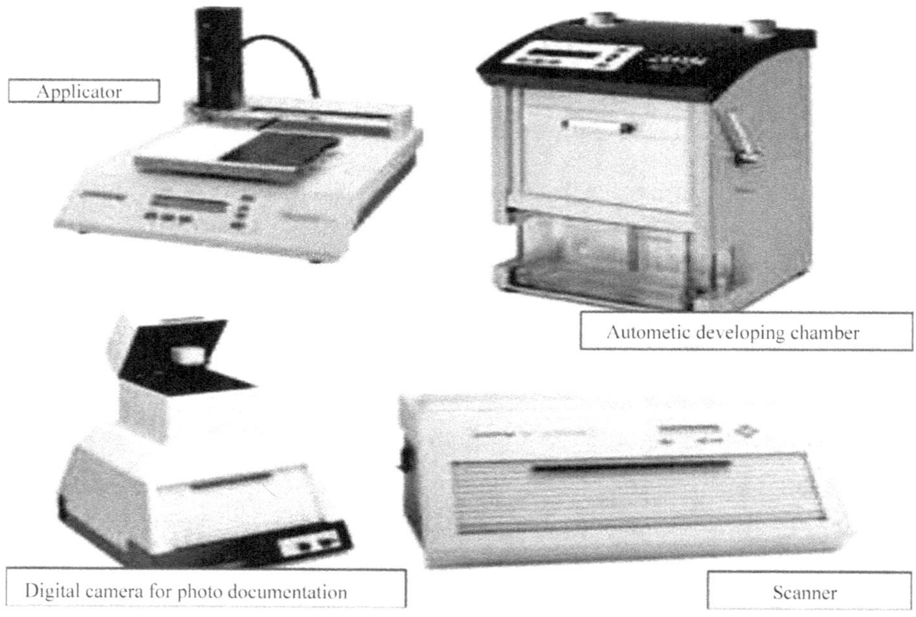

Fig. 5.8 Instrumentation of HPTLC

Column Chromatography

When a column of stationary phase is used for the separation of the phytoconstituents, the technique is called as column chromatography. If the stationary phase used is solid then known as adsorption chromatography while stationary phase used is liquid then known as partition chromatography.

Column adsorption chromatography

In this type of chromatography solid stationary phase and a liquid mobile phase is used and the principle of separation is adsorption. When a mixture of components dissolved in the mobile phase is introduced into the column, the individual components move with different rates depending upon their affinity towards the stationary phase. The component with lesser affinity moves faster and hence it is eluted out of the column first. The compound with more affinity towards the stationary phase moves slower down the column and hence it is eluted later.

Steps involved in column chromatography: Following steps are involved in Column chromatography

1. **Selection of stationary phase:** The adsorbent used as stationary phase should meet following criteria:

   - The particles should have uniform size distribution and have spherical shape. The range of particle size 60-200 μ.

   - Should have high mechanical stability.

   - Should be inert and should not react with the solute or other components.

- Insoluble in mobile phase used.
- It should allow free flow of mobile phase.
- It should be useful for separating for wide variety of components.
- It should be easily available and economic.

2. **Selection of mobile phase:** Mobile phase is very important and they serve several functions. They act as solvent, developer and as eluent. The functions of mobile phase are,
   - To introduce mixture into column as solvent.
   - To develop zone for separation as developing agent.
   - To remove pure component out of the column.
   - Examples of mobile phase, petroleum ether, carbon tetrachloride, cyclohexane.
   - The solvents can be used in pure form or as a mixture of solvents of varying composition

3. **Selection of column:** Generally. the columns are used should not get affected by solvents, acids or alkalies. An ordinary burette can also be used as a column. The column dimensions are important for effective separation. The length: diameter ratio ranges from 10:1 to 30:1, for more efficiency it can be increased up to 100:1.

4. **Preparation of column:** The bottom portion of the column is packed with cotton wool or glass wool or may contain a asbestos pad above which the column of the adsorbent is packed. Sometimes a Whatman filter paper disc can also be used. After packing the column with adsorbent, a similar paper disc is kept on the top, so that the adsorbent layer is not distributed during the introduction of the sample or mobile phase. Column can be packed by two techniques;

   Dry packing technique: In this technique the required quantity of adsorbent is packed in the dry form and the solvent is allowed to flow through the column till equilibrium is reached. In this method the column may not be uniformly packed as air bubbles are entrapped between the solvent and stationary phase.

   Wet packing technique: This is the preferred technique. The required quantity of adsorbent is mixed with the mobile phase solvent in a beaker and then poured into the column. The stationary phase settles uniformly in the column.

5. **Introduction of sample:** The sample to be separated is dissolved in minimum quantity of the mobile phase used for preparing the column. The entire sample is introduced into the column at once. The sample get adsorbed on to the top of the column and then can be separated by elution method.

6. **Selection of development technique (elution):** After the introduction of the sample, by elution techniques, the individual components are separated out from the column. The two techniques are available for development:

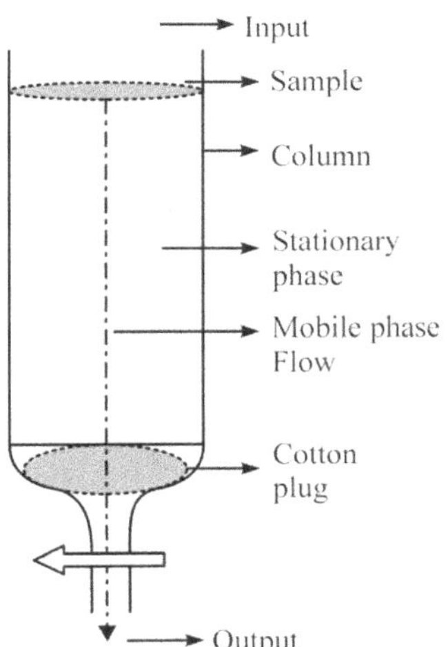

Fig. 5.9 Column Chromatography

Isocratic elution: Iso means same or similar, in this elution technique the same solvent composition or solvent of same polarity are used throughout process of separation. e.g. only chloroform

Gradient elution technique: Gradient means gradually; in this technique solvents of gradually increasing polarity are used during the process of separation. Initially a low polar solvent is used followed by gradually increasing the polarity to a more polar solvent. e.g. Initially chloroform followed by ethyl acetate and then ethanol.

7. **Detection of component:** The colored compounds can be detected by visual observation as different color bands are seen moving down the column and can be collected separately. For colorless components, the technique depends upon the properties of the components e.g.: If components absorb light can be detected by UV or visible detector

8. **Recovery of component:** The recovery can be done by cutting the column into several distinct zones or by using plunger. The best technique is to recover the components by elution. The components are eluate, the solvent called as eluent and the process is elution. The recovery can be done by isocratic or gradient elution or by collecting different fractions of mobile phase of equal volume like 20 ml or by collecting fractions at particular time intervals. The recovered fractions are detected by using different detection techniques.

Applications of Column chromatography

- Separation of mixture of compounds from plant products.

- Used in purification process of isolated compounds from herbal extracts.

- Used for the estimation of drugs in the formulations.

- Used for isolation of phytoconstituents from complex extracts.

- Used for isolation of primary and secondary metabolites of the plants.

High Performance Liquid Chromatography (HPLC)

High-performance liquid chromatography (HPLC) is an instrumental form of liquid chromatography that employs stationary phases consisting of small particles hence achieve more efficient separations than those used in conventional liquid chromatography. It is known by several different names, including high pressure liquid chromatography, because of the high pressures required to force the mobile phase or solvent through the stationary phase, and high-resolution liquid chromatography, because of the good resolution achieved using this technique

HPLC is a form of column chromatography that pumps a sample mixture or analyte in a solvent (known as the mobile phase) at high pressure through a column with chromatographic packing material (stationary phase). The sample is carried by a moving carrier gas stream of helium or nitrogen. HPLC has the ability to separate, and identify compounds that are present in any sample that can be dissolved in a liquid in trace concentrations as low as parts per trillion. Because of this versatility, HPLC is used in a variety of industrial and scientific applications. HPLC operate under the same basic principle; separation of a sample into its components because of the difference in the relative affinities of different components for the mobile phase and the stationary phase used in the separation. The sample gets separated at particular time known as retention time (Rt). Retention time may vary depending on the interaction between the stationary phase, the molecules being analyzed, and the solvent, or solvents used. As the sample passes through the column it interacts between the two phases at different rate, primarily due to different polarities in the components. component that have the least affinity with the stationary phase or more affinity towards the mobile phase will exit the column faster.

There are following types of HPLC, depending upon the phase system (stationary) in the process:

Normal Phase HPLC

This method separates components on the basis of polarity. NP-HPLC uses polar stationary phase and non-polar mobile phase. Therefore, the stationary phase is usually silica and typical mobile phases are hexane, ethyl acetate, chloroform, diethyl ether, and mixtures of any two or more solvents. Polar samples are thus retained on the polar surface of the column packing longer than less polar material.

Reverse phase HPLC

In this type the stationary phase is nonpolar (hydrophobic) in nature, while the mobile phase is a polar liquid, such as mixtures of water and methanol or acetonitrile. It works on the principle of hydrophobic interactions hence the more nonpolar the material is, the longer it will be retained.

Size-exclusion HPLC

The column is filled with material having precisely controlled pore sizes, and the particles are separated according to its their molecular size. Larger molecules are rapidly washed through the column; smaller molecules penetrate inside the porous of the packing particles and elute later.

Ion-Exchange HPLC

The stationary phase has an ionically charged surface of opposite charge to the sample ions. This technique is used almost exclusively with ionic or ionizable samples.

Instrumentation: Main components in an HPLC system include the solvent reservoir, a high-pressure pump, a column, injector system and the detector.

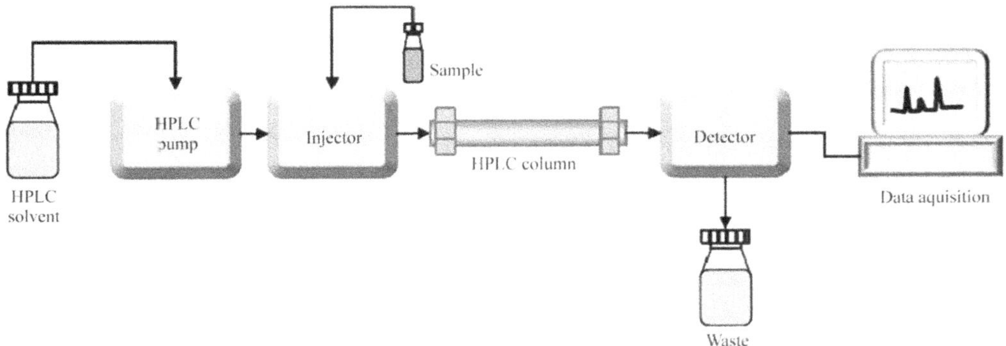

Fig. 5.10 Components of HPLC

Solvent Reservoir: Solvent reservoir consists of mobile phase in a glass reservoir. The mobile phase in HPLC is usually a mixture of polar and non-polar liquids.

Pump: A pump forces the mobile phase from the solvent reservoir through the system's column and detector. Depending on a number of factors including column dimensions, particle size of the stationary phase, the flow rate and composition of the mobile phase, operating pressures of up to 42000 kPa (about 6000 psi) can be generated.

Sample injector: The injector can be a single injection or an automated injection system. An injector for an HPLC system should provide injection of the liquid sample within the range of 0.1-100 ml of volume with high reproducibility and under high pressure (up to 4000 psi).

Columns: Columns are usually made of polished stainless steel, are between 50 and 300 mm long and have an internal diameter of between 2 and 5 mm. They are commonly filled with a stationary phase with a particle size of 3–10 µm.

Detector: The HPLC detector are present at the end of the column to detect the components as they elute from the chromatographic column. Commonly used detectors are UV-spectroscopy, fluorescence, mass-spectrometric and electrochemical detectors.

Data acquisition system: Signals from the detector may be collected on chart recorders or electronic integrators. The computer integrates the response of the detector to each component and places it into a chromatograph that is easy to read and interpret.

Applications of HPLC

- Identification and quantification of the components at very low concentrations.
- Helps in chemical separation and purification of organic compounds.
- Used in quality control of pharmaceuticals and natural products.
- Used to perform the stability studies of the pharmaceuticals and natural products.
- Used to study tablet dissolution.

Gas Chromatography (GC)

It is a common type of chromatography used in analysis for separating and analyzing compounds that can be vaporized without decomposition. Gas chromatography is the process of separating, identifying and quantifying the various compositional elements of a compound. In GC the stationary phase is either in the forms of solid adsorbent (gas-solid chromatography) or liquid on an inert support (gas-liquid chromatography). The mobile phase – It is a chemically inert gas that carries components molecules through the heated column.

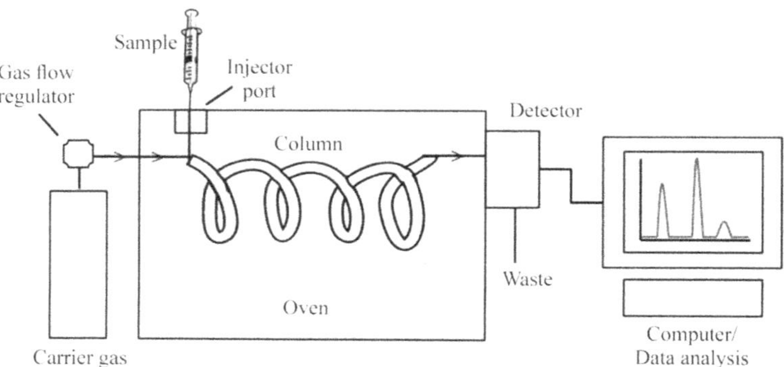

Fig. 5.11 Gas Chromatography

GC is used to separate and detect small molecular weight compounds in the gas phase. The sample is either a gas or a liquid is vaporized in the injection port. The mobile phase for gas chromatography is a carrier gas, generally helium because of its low molecular weight and being chemically inert. The pressure is applied and the mobile phase moves the components through the column. The separation is accomplished using a column coated with a stationary phase.

Applications of GC

- GC analysis is used to calculate the content of a chemical product.

- For measuring toxic substances in soil, air or water and herbal extracts.

- Gas chromatography is used in the analysis of air-borne pollutants, oil spills essential oils in perfume preparation

- GC is very accurate if used properly and can measure picomoles of a substance in a 1 ml liquid sample, or parts-per-billion concentrations in gaseous samples.

- Gas Chromatography is used extensively in forensic science, arson investigation, paint chip analysis, and toxicology cases.

- GC is employed to identify and quantify various biological specimens.

- It is used to separate and detect small molecular weight compounds from volatile oils.

Spectroscopy

Introduction

Spectroscopy is the measurement and interpretation of electromagnetic radiations (EMR) absorbed or emitted when the molecule or atoms or ions of a sample move from one energy state to another energy state. This change may be from ground state to excited state or excited state to ground state. At ground state energy of a molecule is the sum total of rotational, vibrational and electronic energies. In short spectroscopy measures the changes in rotational, vibrational or electronic energies.

Classification of spectroscopy

1. Based on whether the study is made at atomic or molecular level:

    I. Atomic spectroscopy: In this type the changes in energy at atomic level are studied. e.g. Atomic absorption spectroscopy.

    II. Molecular spectroscopy: In this type the changes in energy at molecular level are studied. e.g. InfraRed spectroscopy, ultra violet spectroscopy.

2. Based on whether the study is of absorption or emission of EMR:

    I. Absorption spectroscopy: Here absorption of radiation is being studied. e.g. Atomic absorption spectroscopy

    II. Emission spectroscopy: Here emission of radiation is being studied. e.g. flame photometry, fluorimetry.

3. Based on electronic or magnetic level studies:
   I. Electronic spectroscopy: Here study is done using EMR only without the influence of magnetic field. e.g. UV spectroscopy, fluorimetry
   II. Magnetic spectroscopy: Here the study is done using EMR under the influence of magnetic field.

UV/Visible Spectroscopy

UV spectroscopy is type of absorption spectroscopy in which light of ultra-violet region (200-400 nm) is absorbed by the molecule which results in the excitation of the electrons from the ground state to higher energy state. Basically, spectroscopy is related to the interaction of light with matter.

As light is absorbed by matter, the result is an increase in the energy content of the atoms or molecules. When ultraviolet radiations are absorbed, this results in the excitation of the electrons from the ground state towards a higher energy state. Molecules containing π-electrons or non-bonding electrons (n-electrons) can absorb energy in the form of ultraviolet light to excite these electrons to higher anti-bonding molecular orbitals.

The more easily excited the electrons, the longer the wavelength of light it can absorb. There are four possible types of transitions and they can be ordered as follows:

$$\sigma-\sigma^* > n-\sigma^* > \pi-\pi^* > n-\pi^*$$

The absorption of ultraviolet light by a chemical compound will produce a distinct spectrum which aids in the identification of the compound.

Instrumentation

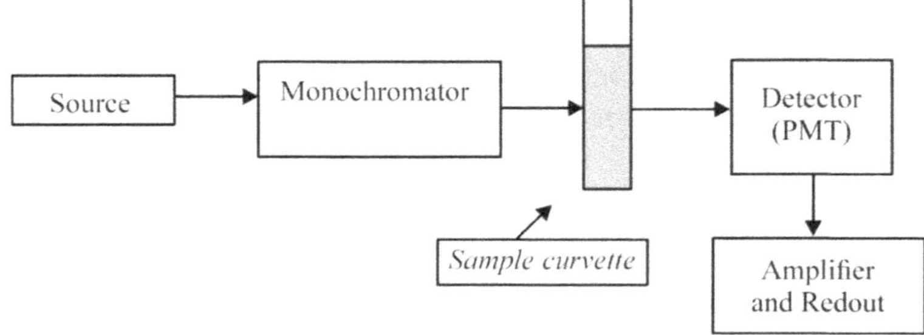

Fig. 5.12 Instrumentation of UV spectroscopy

Light Source: Tungsten filament lamps and Hydrogen-Deuterium lamps are most widely used and suitable light source as they cover the whole UV region.

Monochromator: Monochromator generally is composed of entrance slit, dispersing prisms and exit slit. The radiation emitted from the primary source is dispersed with the help of rotating prisms. The various wavelengths of the light source which are separated by the prism are then selected by the slits. The beam selected by the slit is monochromatic and further divided into two beams with the help of another prism.

Sample and reference cells: One of the two divided beams is passed through the sample solution and second beam is passé through the reference solution. Both sample and reference solution are contained in the cells. These cells are made of either silica or quartz. Glass can't be used for the cells as it also absorbs light in the UV region.

Detector: Generally, two photocells serve the purpose of detector in UV spectroscopy. One of the photocells receives the beam from sample cell and second detector receives the beam from the reference. The intensity of the radiation from the reference cell is stronger than the beam of sample cell. This results in the generation of pulsating or alternating currents in the photocells.

Amplifier: The alternating current generated in the photocells is transferred to the amplifier. The main purpose of amplifier is to amplify the signals many times so we can get clear and recordable signals.

Recorder: Most of the time amplifier is coupled to a recorder which is connected to the computer. Computer stores all the data generated and produces the spectrum of the desired compound.

Applications of UV spectroscopy

- Useful in structural elucidation of organic compounds.
- It is one of the best methods for determination of impurities in organic molecules.
- It is used in molecular weight determination of isolated compounds.
- It helps to distinct *Cis* and *Trans* isomerism.
- It helps to study conjugation effects.

Infra-Red Spectroscopy

Infrared Spectroscopy is the analysis of *infrared* light interacting with a molecule. This can be analyzed in three ways by measuring absorption, emission and reflection. It is used to determine the functional groups in molecules. The spectra of a molecule arises in IR region ($12500 \text{ cm}^{-1} - 50 \text{ cm}^{-1}$) due to the absorption of energy and transition occurs between different vibrational levels. Hence it is called vibration spectroscopy. All types of molecules cannot interact with IR radiation. Only those molecules which exhibit change in dipole moment during a vibration can exhibit IR spectra. The IR spectral region at $1400 \text{ cm}^{-1} - 700 \text{ cm}^{-1}$ gives rich, intense and clear absorption bands for all functional groups in the organic compounds. This region is called **finger–print region.** It is used to identify the functional group present in the organic compound, Identify the molecule and find out the characteristics of the molecule.

The IR spectral region at $4000 \text{ cm}^{-1} - 600 \text{ cm}^{-1}$ gives intense absorption bands associated with bending and stretching vibrations of particular functional group in organic compounds. This region is called **group frequency region.** It is used to identify the types of functional groups present in organic molecules.

Instrumentation

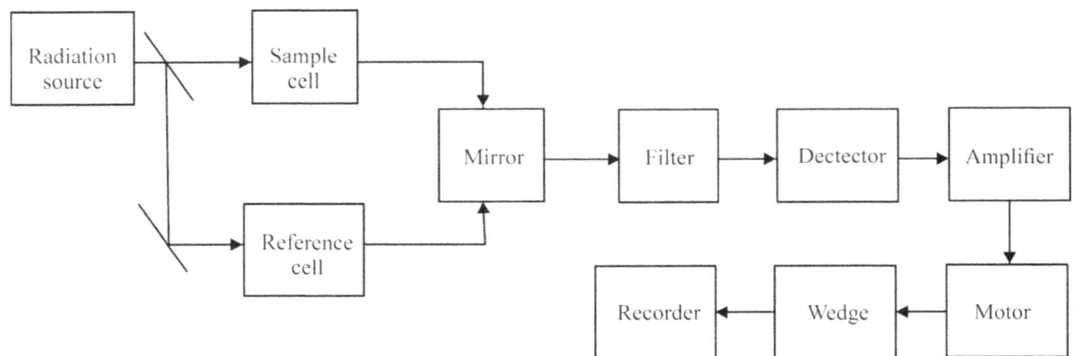

Fig. 5.13 Block diagram of IR spectrophotometer

Radiation source: The Nernst glower (Oxides of Zr, Y and Er) is heated to 1500°C to give IR radiation, which is used as radiation source.

Optical prism: It is also called mirror, which is used to reflect the radiation on filter.

Filter: It is also called monochromator, which sent the individual frequencies to the detector.

Amplifier: It amplifies the current received from the detector.

Motor: It drives the wedge.

Recorder: It draws the IR spectrum, based on the movement of wedge.

Working: The IR radiation from radiation source is splitted into two equal half beams; one half is passed into the sample cell and another half is passed into the reference cell containing solvent respectively. Then these beams are fall on the mirror and reflected to the monochromator, where the selective radiation is sent to the detector. The radiation received by the detector is converted into current. It is amplified and coupled to the motor which drives a wedge. Based on the movement of the wedge the recorder draws the absorption bands on the chart. Finally, we get a spectrum as a graph of Transmittance verses wave number from the IR spectrophotometer.

Applications

1. It is used to identify the presence of functional groups in organic compounds.
2. It is used to detect the presence of impurities in organic compounds, by comparing the IR spectra of the pure (shows actual absorption bands) and impure (shows extra absorption bands) compounds.
3. It is used to distinguish inter and intra molecular hydrogen bonding in organic compounds.
4. It is used to study the molecular symmetry, dipole moment, structure, bond angle and bond length, etc. of various organic and inorganic compounds.
5. It is used to distinguish positional isomers of organic compounds.
6. It is used in rapid quantitative analysis of mixture of compounds.
7. It is used to study the kinetics of a reaction.

Mass Spectroscopy

Mass spectrometry (MS) is an analytical technique that measures the mass-to-charge ratio of ions. The results are generally presented as a mass spectrum, a plot of intensity as a function of the mass-to-charge ratio. Mass spectrum is also called as a positive ion spectrum. The mass spectra can be obtained by two steps;

- Conversion of neutral molecule into a charged molecule, preferably positively charged molecule

- Separation of the positively charged fragments formed, based on their masses by using electrical or magnetic field or both.

Instrumentation

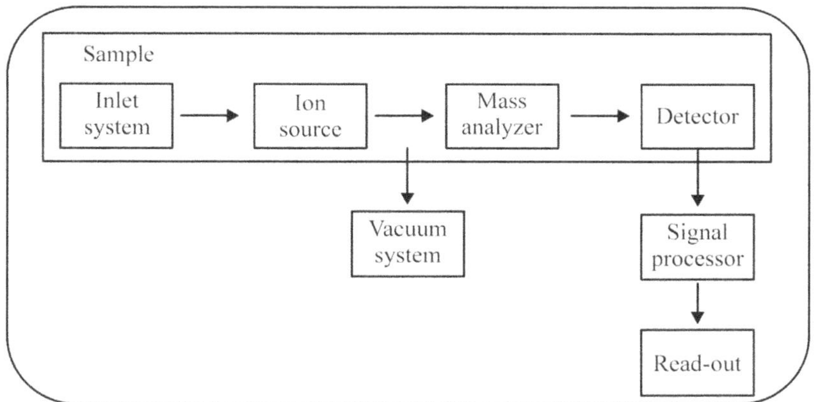

Fig. 5.14 Instrumentation of mass spectrophotometer

With all the above components, a mass spectrometer should always perform the following processes:

- Ions are produced from the sample in the ionization source.

- These ions are separated according to their mass-to-charge ratio in the mass analyzer.

- Eventually, the selected ions are fragmented and the fragments are analyzed in a second analyzer.

- The ions emerging from the last analyzer are detected and their abundance can be measured with the detector that converts the ions into electrical signals.

- The signals are processed from the detector that are transmitted to the computer and control the instrument using feedback.

Applications of Mass spectroscopy

- MS is used in structure elucidation by using nitrogen rule, peak matching, fragmentation pattern of compounds.

- For detection of impurities present in isolated phytoconstituents.

- MS is used in Quantitative analysis of phytoconstituents
- To study metabolism of natural products.

Nuclear Magnetic Resonance Spectroscopy

Nuclear Magnetic Resonance Spectroscopy is commonly known as NMR spectroscopy. It is based on the measurement of absorption of electromagnetic radiation by the nuclei of the atom in the radio frequency region of roughly 4 to 900 MHz under the influence of strong magnetic field. NMR is the most powerful tool for structural elucidation of the compound. The principal behind the NMR is that many nuclei have spin and all nuclei are electrically charged. Under the influence of the magnetic field, energy transfers from the base energy to a higher energy level. This energy transfers takes place a wavelength that corresponds to the radiofrequencies and when the spin returns to its base level, energy is emitted at the same frequency.

Instrumentation

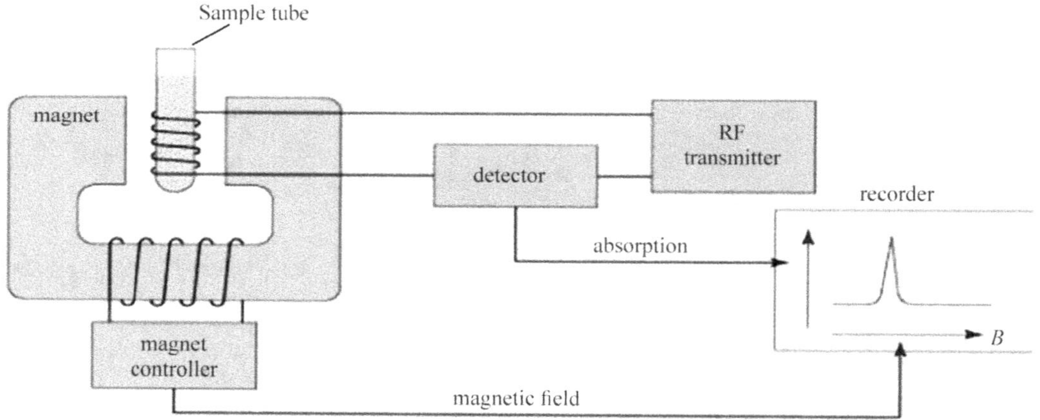

Fig. 5.15 Instrumentation of NMR

1. **Sample holder:** Glass tube with 8.5 cm long, 0.3 cm in diameter.
2. **Permanent magnet:** It provides homogeneous magnetic field at 60-100 MHZ.
3. **Magnetic coils:** These coils induce magnetic field when current flows through them.
4. **Sweep generator:** To produce the equal amount of magnetic field pass through the sample.
5. **Radio frequency transmitter:** A radio transmitter coil transmitter that produces a short powerful pulse of radio waves.
6. **Radio frequency receiver:** A radio receiver coil that detects radio frequencies emitted as nuclei relax to a lower energy level.
7. **Recorder:** A computer that analyses and record the data.

Working: The sample is placed in a magnetic field and the NMR signal is produced by excitation of the nuclei sample with radio waves into nuclear magnetic resonance, which is detected with sensitive radio receivers. The intramolecular magnetic field around an atom in a molecule changes the resonance frequency, thus provides details of the electronic structure of a molecule and its individual functional groups

Applications of NMR spectroscopy

- It is an analytical chemistry technique used in quality control.
- It is used in research for determining the content and purity of a sample as well as its molecular structure.
- NMR spectroscopy is routinely used to study chemical structure using simple one-dimensional techniques. Two-dimensional techniques are used to determine the structure of more complicated molecules.
- Used in structural determination of proteins.
- Solid state NMR spectroscopy is used to determine the molecular structure of solids.

Electrophoresis

Electrophoresis is a physical method of analysis which involves separation of the compounds that are capable of acquiring electric charge in conducting electrodes. Electrophoresis may be defined as the migration of the charged particle through a solution under the influence of an external electrical field. Ions that are suspended between two electrodes tend to travel towards the electrode that bears opposite charges.

Types of electrophoresis: The electrophoresis can be categorized into many types. Few of them are mentioned here.

- **Paper Electrophoresis:** This technique is useful for the separation of small charged molecules such as amino acids and small proteins. A strip of filter paper is moistened with buffer and the ends of the strip are immersed into buffer reservoirs containing the electrodes. The samples are spotted in the center of the paper, high voltage is applied and the spots migrate according to their charges. After electrophoresis, the separated components can be detected by a variety of staining techniques, depending upon their chemical identity. This method also useful for determination of protein isoelectric point. It has very useful application in blood cell separation.

- **Affinity Electrophoresis:** The methods are based on changes in the ectrophoretic pattern of molecules through bio specific interaction or complex formation.

- **Capillary Electrophoresis:** It is also known as Capillary Zone Electrophoresis (CZE). This can be used to separate ionic species by their charge and frictional forces and hydrodynamic radius. It can be performed in a capillary format. A typical system consists of two reservoirs and a capillary filled with a buffer solution.

- **Dielectrophoresis (DEP):** It is a phenomenon in which a force is exerted on a dielectric particle when it is subjected to non-uniform electric field. This force doesn't require the particle to be charged. All particles exhibit dielectrophoretic activity in the presence of electric fields.

- **DNA Electrophoresis:** It is an analytical technique used to separate DNA fragments by size.

- **Gel Electrophoresis:** It refers to using a gel as an anticonvective medium and/or sieving medium during electrophoresis. Gel electrophoresis is most commonly used for separation of biological macromolecules such as DNA, RNA or proteins. It refers to the movement of charged particles in an electric field. Gel suppress the thermal convection caused by application of the electric field, and can act as a sieving medium, retarding the passage of molecules, gel also can simply to serve to maintain the finished separation, so that a post electrophoresis stain can be applied.

- **Immunoelectrophoresis:** It is also called as Gamma Globulin Electrophoresis or Immunoglobulin Electrophoresis, is a method of determining the blood levels of three major immunoglobulins: IgM, IgG, IgA. it is a powerful analytical technique with high resolving power as it combines separation of antigens by electrophoresis with immuno diffusion against an antiserum.

- **Pulsed Field Gel Electrophoresis (PFGE):** It is a technique used for the separation of large DNA molecules by applying an electric field that periodically changes direction to a gel matrix.

Application of Electrophoresis

- Electrophoresis is mainly used for the separation of ionizable substances by using buffers of different pH and ionic strength.

- Separation of amino acids.

- Separation of lipoproteins in serum (in case of hyperlipidemia).

- Separation of enzymes from blood.

- For the separation of ions containing same electrophoretic mobility, Isotachophoresis is used to separate the ions by gradient pH application.

- Dielectrophoresis can be used to manipulate, transport, separate and sort different types of particles.

- Separation of alkaloids and antibiotics in different samples can be carried out.

- Used for DNA separation and analysis.

Probable Questions

Long answer questions

1. Define extraction. Explain in detail the conventional methods of extractions.
2. Explain in detail continuous hot extraction. Write its advantages and disadvantages.
3. Write detail note on Microwave assisted extraction (MAE).
4. Define Chromatography. Explain in detail steps involved in TLC.
5. Define and classify chromatography. Write brief note on HPTLC.
6. Explain in detail High Performance Liquid Chromatography.
7. Explain in detail electrophoresis and its types.

Short answer questions

1. Write short note on Soxhlet extractor.
2. Explain in brief supercritical fluid extraction.
3. Define and classify spectroscopy. Explain principle of UV spectrophotometer.
4. Write short note on IR spectroscopy.
5. Write applications of Gas chromatography in phytochemical analysis.
6. Write applications of electrophoresis.
7. Define maceration and percolation. Explain percolator in brief.

Very Short answer questions

1. Define extraction. What are the factors affecting extraction efficiency.
2. Write the principle of SFE.
3. Write the principle of TLC/HPTLC.
4. Explain in brief the principle of GC.
5. Explain in brief principle of NMR Spectroscopy.
6. Define the terms *Rf* value, RPHPLC and gel electrophoresis.